THE NATURAL PROSTATE CURE

THIRD EDITION

Other Health Books
by Roger Mason

THE NATURAL PROSTATE CURE

THIRD EDITION

A Practical Guide to Using Diet and Lifestyle for a Healthy Prostate

ROGER MASON

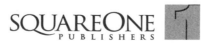

SQUAREONE
PUBLISHERS

The information and advice contained in this book are based upon the research and the personal and professional experiences of the author. They are not intended as a substitute for consulting with a healthcare professional. The publisher and author are not responsible for any adverse effects or consequences resulting from the use of any of the suggestions or procedures discussed in this book. All matters pertaining to your physical health should be supervised by a healthcare professional. It is a sign of wisdom, not cowardice, to seek a second or third opinion.

Square One Publishers
115 Herricks Road
Garden City Park, NY 11040
(516) 535-2010 (877) 900-Book

ISBN 978-0-7570-0476-6 (pb)

Printed in the United States of America

10   9   8   7   6   5   4   3   2   1

Contents

"If people let the government decide what foods they eat and what medicines they take, their bodies will soon be in as sorry a state as the souls who live under tyranny."

—THOMAS JEFFERSON

Introduction

Doctors are still castrating men with chemicals instead of surgery! This insanity has to stop. There is no reason for men to continue to be senselessly poisoned, irradiated, and butchered by the medical profession. Treating the symptoms of prostate disease, instead of the causes, has very drastic results—including diapers and impotence for the rest of a man's life. Prostate problems can be cured naturally with a healthy diet, proven supplements, natural hormones, exercise, fasting, and by avoiding prescription drugs and dropping any bad habits. *Diet and lifestyle cure disease.*

This book contains the distillation of forty years of prostate research. All of the information has been refined and written in plain English. In the last fifteen years, it has been rewritten and expanded fourteen times. This is the most informative, comprehensive, and researched book on prostate health in the world. Over two million men in most every country have now read *The Natural Prostate Cure.* By taking responsibility for their conditions, men can cure themselves naturally with the information herein.

The prostate is an integral part of the reproductive system, so any prostate-related illness can cause serious sexual performance problems. Men may encounter three main issues:

1

infection (prostatitis), enlargement (benign prostate hypertrophy, or BPH), and cancer.

By the age of fifty, three out of four men already have enlarged prostates, and one in three men have cancer cells in their prostates. This, clearly, is not an "old man's disease" at all. By the time they reach the age of seventy-five, an astounding three out of four men in America have cancer cells in their prostate. It is the leading form of male cancer. The symptoms are very obvious—difficulty in urination, inability to empty the bladder completely, pain during sex or urination, sexual dysfunction, and, especially, the need to urinate in the middle of the night. All of these are classic symptoms of prostate problems.

The real cure comes from changing your diet and lifestyle. Treat the very cause of your problem. Diet is everything. Natural health includes proper diet, proven supplements, natural hormone balance, weekly fasting, regular exercise, refusing prescription drugs, and ending negative habits (such as drinking coffee). Holistic medicine treats the whole person instead of just alleviating the symptoms of a disease. Think "whole body health," and not just "prostate." Symptoms reflect the underlying causes of our illnesses, and are harbingers of even worse health in the future. Always treat the cause of your illness, not just the symptoms.

1. Diet

iet is everything! Diet cures disease. A natural, whole food diet is the most important thing you need in order to get well and stay well. Diet and lifestyle cure illness. By eating a traditional whole grain-based, low-fat diet, you can actually eliminate prostate infection, enlargement, and even cancer.

If you doubt this, read actor Dirk Benedict's book *Confessions of a Kamikaze Cowboy*. Dirk was diagnosed with prostate cancer in his early thirties, and the doctors wanted to castrate him. That didn't appeal to him much, so he decided to go on a *macrobiotic* (Greek for "prolonging life") diet of whole grains, beans, vegetables, soups, salads, seafood, and fruits. He quit eating red meat, poultry, eggs, dairy products, sweeteners of all kinds, refined foods, preservatives, and the like. After only seven months, Dirk knew he was well. He is now seventy-three, still active, healthy, happy, youthful, vibrant, the father of two grown sons, and a grandfather. If Dirk had listened to his doctors, he would have died many years ago as a sexless eunuch in diapers.

Eating a whole grain-based diet is an essential part of getting well. *Diet is everything.* Supplements, hormones, exercise, and fasting are all secondary. When you are eating well, these additions are very powerful and make your recovery rapid. Without whole, healthy, natural food, it doesn't matter what else you do; you're just not going to get well. *Diet cures disease.*

3

THE SECRET TO GOOD HEALTH

We've all heard of people, like the rural Okinawans, who live very long lives and have low disease rates. Well, you don't have to live in a remote farming village and give up all the conveniences of the modern world to live a long and healthy life. You just have to change your diet and lifestyle. Such long-lived people eat whole grains, beans, vegetables, seafood, local fruits, and very little, if any, meat, poultry, eggs, or dairy products. Generally, their fat intake makes up only about 10 percent of their diet, and consists of mainly vegetable oils, rather than saturated animal fats.

There are a variety of good books on macrobiotics in print now. Please read some of them. For optimum health, your diet should be based on whole grains and beans. Whole grains are the staff of life. Most all vegetables are fine, but the nightshade family (potatoes, tomatoes, peppers, eggplant) should be avoided. Also avoid vegetables containing excess oxalic acid (spinach, rhubarb, red chard). Any bean or legume is fine, and there are dozens of varieties. Beans are good food. Local fruit can be eaten in moderation, especially in summer. Seafood can also be eaten in moderation if you do not want to be a vegetarian, as long as you are not allergic to it. Nuts are very high in fat (generally 90 percent fat calories), and should only be used as a garnish. Healthy soups and salads are good additions to your meals if they are made with macrobiotic ingredients. Avoid red meat, poultry, eggs, and dairy products of all kinds. Do not eat refined foods, processed foods, or sweeteners of any kind (including honey). Avoid tropical foods such as citrus, pineapples, mangos, and coconuts (all of which are meant for tropical populations in their native environments). Tropical races living in warm climates can, and should, eat such foods, of course.

One of the best studies on prostate health was conducted at Loma Linda University (*American Journal of Epidemiology* v 120, 1982). Researchers studied 6,735 men for what they ate. The men had a direct relation between the animal foods they ate and their rates of prostate cancer. They also had the same direct relation with obesity. The more meat or poultry they ate, the more cancer they got. The more milk and cheese they ate, the more cancer they got. The more eggs they ate, the more cancer they got. The really interesting thing about these findings is that men who ate all four of these food groups had extremely high prostate cancer rates. These foods work synergistically to support malignancies. This study, among others, proves the basic thesis that an excess of dietary saturated animal fat and protein is the underlying cause of prostate disease. As you will see in the next chapter, an abundance of statistical data strongly supports this theory.

THE STAFF OF LIFE

Whole grains should be the basis of your daily food. This includes brown rice, whole grain breads, whole wheat pasta, corn, barley, rye, millet, oats, spelt, buckwheat, and quinoa. People who eat whole grains are healthier, live longer, and are less likely to develop diseases of all kinds. Americans only eat about one percent whole grains, when they should be eating at least 50 percent. The fact that we eat a mere one percent of whole grains says everything about our diet.

At the University of California in San Diego (*Integrative Cancer Therapies* v 5, 2006), progressive doctors gave prostate cancer patients a low-fat, whole grain-based diet including lots of vegetables for six months. These men improved remarkably, and lived much longer than the patients receiving the standard medical treatment. At the University of California in Los Angeles (*American Journal of Clinical Nutrition* v 86, 2007), men were put on a vegetarian form of the Pritikin diet, which is based in low-fat, high-fiber food. Their insulin levels fell dramatically, and their risk factors for prostate cancer were greatly reduced.

Again at the University of California in Los Angeles (*Recent Results in Cancer Research* v 166, 2005), studies showed that metabolic syndrome (high blood sugar and insulin resistance) correlated with prostate cancer. Men given a low-fat diet and exercise lowered their insulin levels greatly. At Queen's University in Canada (*International Journal of Cancer* v 116, 2005), doctors studied the dietary patterns of men. Those who included whole grains and vegetables in their daily fare had far lower prostate cancer rates than the ones who ate meat, milk, sugar, and refined grains.

Dean Ornish's Preventive Medicine Research Institute (*Journal of the American Dietetic Association* v 105, 2005) has been working with prostate cancer patients. They gave these patients a low-fat vegan diet with very impressive results: The patients lived longer and had much better health. Dean and his associates at the University of California in San Francisco (*Journal of Urology* v 174, 2005) fed prostate cancer patients a vegan diet for one year. Patients also took a few basic supplements and exercised regularly. The men refused all traditional medical treatments including surgery, drugs, and radiation. This simple regimen slowed down, and even reversed, the cancer growth. If Dean would just go a little further and adopt macrobiotics, proven supplements, natural hormones, and fasting, these men could be cured of cancer instead of just living longer.

An entire book, *Whole Grain Foods in Health and Disease* (2002), is devoted to the health benefits of eating whole, unprocessed, unrefined grains. The authors found that people who eat whole grains are far less likely to get cancer, especially prostate or breast cancer. The books *The China Study* and *The Okinawan Plan* are also very good.

Americans eat very few fresh (or frozen) green and yellow vegetables. Asians, especially rural Asians, eat the most vegetables, and prepare them in the most delicious ways. They also tend to consume a great deal of soy products. Refer to the following section "The Power of Soy" to learn how soy can be especially helpful in reducing prostate cancer rates. You want to eat more fresh (or even frozen vegetables, since they actually have more nutrients) every day. Johns Hopkins University (*American Journal of Clinical Nutrition* v 85, 2007) studied over 30,000 men. They found a strong correlation between the large amount of vegetables the men ate and the small number of men who developed prostate disease. At the Negri Institute in Italy, doctors found the same phenomenon (*International Journal of Cancer* v 109, 2004). Vegetables and vegetable fiber protected men from prostate cancer.

The Power of Soy

Soy foods are very effective in reducing the rates of various cancers, especially prostate and breast cancer. Asian cultures eat quite a lot of these soy foods in various forms. The longest-lived people on earth, the Okinawans, eat the most soy of anyone, with a caloric intake of 12 percent. It is unrealistic and impractical to ask Westerners to do this for several reasons. Boiled soybeans, per se, just don't taste very good. Tofu is not a whole food, nor is it very nutritious. Most people have never heard of tempeh, seitan, or natto, and have little interest in eating them. Soy sauce is merely a condiment. A little miso goes a long way, but it is basically used only in soup. How much soy flour can you really add to your baked goods? Soy milk, however, is a realistic way to increase your soy intake. Soy isoflavones, as a supplement, are also a practical option, and are recommended in Chapter 3.

CUTTING OUT FAT

Meat, poultry, eggs, and dairy contain heavy amounts of saturated fat, which is the main dietary cause of prostate and other cancers. Saturated animal fat (and protein) is the basic cause of prostate disease. Vegetable oils should only be used in moderation at 10 to 20 percent total calories. All fats must be limited. At

Wake Forest University (*Prostate* v 63, 2005), it was found that the phytanic acid found in red meat and dairy products definitely contributes to cancer of the prostate. The National Cancer Institute studied the diets of 29,361 men (*Cancer Research* v 65, 2005) and showed that red meat is definitely a prostate cancer promoter. In general, animal foods promote disease due to the fat, protein, and cholesterol in them.

Dairy milk (including low-fat milk) contains large amounts of lactose and casein, regardless of the fat content. The protein casein has been shown to promote cancer. Drinking milk has repeatedly been shown to correlate with prostate disease (*Prostate* v 33, 1997 and *Science* v 285, 1999). Yogurt actually has twice the amount of lactose, since dried milk powder is added to thicken it. People of all races, especially blacks and Asians, lose their ability to digest lactose when the body stops producing lactase, the enzyme necessary to digest dairy, after the age of three. Adding lactase tablets to your dairy foods or buying lactose-reduced milk will not solve the problem. Instead, use soy, almond, oat, flax, or rice milk, whether refrigerated or in aseptic shelf packs, as these items are now commonly available in grocery stores. Visit the website NotMilk.com to learn more. Take dairy out of your life.

The Fox Chase Cancer Center (*American Journal Clinical Nutrition* v 81, 2005) has stated that "dairy intake may increase prostate cancer risk." The National Institute of Health (*International Journal of Cancer* v 120, 2007) found that "total dairy intake was also positively associated with risk of prostate cancer." According to the Inserm in Paris (*British Journal of Nutrition* v 95, 2006), "Our data support the hypothesis that dairy products have a harmful effect with respect to the risk of prostate cancer." At the University of Bristol (the *British Journal of Cancer* v 88, 2003), they found intake of dairy foods raised IGF-1 (insulin-like growth factor 1) levels, which in turn raised the rates of prostate, breast, and other cancers. The proof is overwhelming: Dairy intake causes prostate disease.

CUTTING OUT SUGAR

High blood sugar and insulin levels and insulin resistance have been correlated with prostate disease. Americans eat about 160 pounds of various unneeded sweeteners in their food every year. Asians and Africans, who have the lowest prostate disease rates, eat only a fraction of that amount. Excess sugar consumption of any kind can cause high insulin, insulin resistance, high blood sugar, metabolic syndrome, and diabetes.

Sugar is sugar is sugar, whether it is honey, maple syrup, brown sugar, "raw" sugar, molasses, sorghum syrup, cane syrup, dextrose, fructose, maltose, fruit syrup, amazake, fruit juice, fruit concentrate, invert sugar, corn syrup, agave, dried fruit, or any other form of sweetener. This includes stevia, sucralose, and other sugar substitutes, since they act like sugar in our bodies. It's always good for a laugh to see someone in a health food store paying several dollars for a small bag of "raw" sugar or agave nectar, thinking that this is somehow different, not really sugar, and not really bad for them.

ENDING BAD HABITS

Bad habits such as smoking, drinking alcohol, using recreational drugs, and drinking coffee or energy drinks obviously worsen your health. Smoking ages people dramatically. More than one drink of alcohol a day causes poor health in general. Coffee and energy drinks are outright addictions. The use of various recreational drugs, addictive or not, is also epidemic. Lack of exercise is another basic cause of bad health overall.

Obesity is definitely correlated with prostate conditions (*Urology* v 58, 2001). Being overweight strongly increases your chances of getting prostate disease. Exercise is vital for good health, especially if you are trying to recover from an illness. Study after study shows how being overweight causes higher rates of every known illness (except osteoporosis). Does anything correlate *positively* with prostate health? Yes, whole grains, fiber, and vegetable intake do, as do slimness, eating fewer calories, and low-fat diets.

LESS IS MORE

It is very important to eat fewer calories. Americans eat about twice the calories, twice the protein, and more than five times the fat they need. Yes, we eat for two people. *Calorie restriction is the most proven and effective way to extend your life span.* Nothing else has been shown to make you live longer and live better than eating fewer calories. Long-term clinical studies with animals, including monkeys, have proven this fact. Moreover, short-term human studies also have verified the benefits of eating fewer calories. The only author on this subject is Roy Walford, who wrote *The 120-Year Diet* and *Maximum Lifespan*. (Unfortunately, he went in a different direction with *Beyond the 120-Year Diet*.)

The average man needs only about 1,800 calories a day, and a woman only needs about 1,200 calories. You can easily eat just two meals a day, instead of three. You can also fast (fasting means *only* consuming water) one day a week by skipping breakfast and lunch on a specified day. Just eat dinner on a given night, and don't eat again until dinner the next night. Longer fasts may be done periodically for more powerful effects.

Doctors at the University of Wisconsin (*Prostate* v 36, 1998) improved the immunity of prostate glands in rats by merely lowering their caloric intake. Other doctors at the university showed that lowering the calorie intake of mice altered their entire genetic aging profile and allowed them to live much longer, with greatly enhanced immunity.

Researchers in Takatsuki, Japan (*Takeda Kenkyushoho* v 53, 1994) actually reduced the prostate weights of rats by simply giving them less food. Doctors at the University of Umea in Sweden (the *Journal of Cancer* v 58, 1986) gave rats with prostate cancer less food, inhibiting the growth of their tumors. Long-term studies on primates about calorie restriction have shown excellent results. At the Hutchinson Cancer Center (*Cancer*

Epidemiology v 11, 2002), men who ate the least calories had only half the prostate cancer of the control group. This, in addition to eating the right foods, is the most effective means you can use to lengthen and improve the quality of your life. In 2018, we now have real human studies.

CONCLUSION

Paleolithic ("Paleo"), glycemic, gluten free, and ketogenic diets are still popular, unfortunately. The Atkins and South Beach Diets went by the wayside after Dr. Atkins died prematurely from chronic heart disease. All these diets avoid whole grains, but include large amounts of animal foods.

Whole grains should be the very basis of your diet. Ketosis is, in fact, a pathological state in which the body is literally starving for complex carbohydrates. The "glycemic index" classifies whole grains, such as brown rice and oatmeal, as being identical in effect to simple sugars such as cake or candy. The standard of reference is white bread! That is preposterous!

Start using brown rice instead of white rice or potatoes. Eat whole wheat pasta instead of refined white pasta. Find 100 percent whole grain breads without preservatives. Buy 100 percent whole grain hot and cold cereals without sugar. *Make whole grains the basis of each meal.* The words "carbohydrates" or "carbs" are basically meaningless. Eating simple sugars and refined grains should certainly be avoided. Whole grains are literally the "staff of life," and always have been throughout history. Whole grains have been our staple food since mankind first learned to cultivate crops. Make whole grains and beans the very basis of your daily food.

2. Fats

The saturated animal fats in red meat, poultry, eggs, and dairy products seem to hold a hypnotic attraction for many people. The fad diets, including paleo, ketogenic, and gluten-free, emphasize animal foods instead of whole grains and beans. Americans eat about 42 percent fat calories! Most all of these are saturated animal fats, which are the most harmful.

Common sense tells us that high–fat diets are bad for us. They cause obesity, diabetes, heart and artery disease, promote various cancers, and shorten our lives. Studies for the last fifty years have proven repeatedly that high-fat diets cause disease, poor health, and early death. Eating meat, poultry, eggs, and dairy products as staples is obviously the road to Hell. It seems that people just want an excuse to eat high fat foods and rationalize bad habits. People in all European countries eat about 40 percent fat calories, most of which are saturated. The more affluent a society is, the richer the diet is in animal foods and saturated fats—and the higher the disease rates. Ironically, prosperity brings poor health.

HIGH FAT INTAKE AND PROSTATE DISEASE

Countless published studies show high fat intake is correlated with every disease known. This is not debatable. We have used some of the older studies because they are actually better than the modern ones. High fat intake is especially correlated with prostate disease in men and breast disease in women—the two leading types of cancers.

There are far too many studies to even begin to list that show the relation of fat intake, especially saturated animal fat, to prostate disease. Please take a long look at Figure 2.1 on page 15; it will leave no doubt in your mind that *saturated fat intake is the major cause of prostate cancer-related deaths*. The figure is based on the diets of literally billions of people and just cannot be contested. The diets of men in countries like China and Japan get only about 10 percent of their calories from fat. These people suffer only a fraction of the prostate cancer-related deaths that we have in America. If fifteen men per 100,000 die from prostate cancer in the United States, fewer than two men per 100,000 die in China. Point made.

THE TRUTH ABOUT FAT

Hydrogenated fats are the worst. They do not exist in nature, and our bodies just cannot deal with them. Eating vegetable oils is simply a lesser evil. The idea that there are "good fats" and "bad fats" is an illusion. All fats should be limited, including vegetable oils. The less fat you eat, the better! The less fat you eat, the healthier you will be, and the longer you will live. When Asian or African men move to the United States, but maintain their traditional diets, they still get almost no prostate disease of any kind. This is called a "migration study," and the results are inarguable.

The only exception to the fat "rule" is when a supplement of 1 to 2 g per day of flaxseed oil is taken. Flax is a much better choice than fish oil for a lot of reasons. Flax oil contains the valuable omega-3 fatty acid, alpha linolenic acid. Flax oil has a mere nine calories per gram—an insignificant daily calorie intake. Our dietary ratio of omega-6 fatty acids to omega-3s is too high. We eat few foods that contain the omega-3s. Buy and keep your flax oil refrigerated.

Nuts can be eaten in moderation as a garnish. Nuts are usually about 90 percent fat calories, so they cannot be used as a main source of food. Toasted nuts add lots of flavor to your basic foods. Peanuts are allergenic tropical legumes, not nuts.

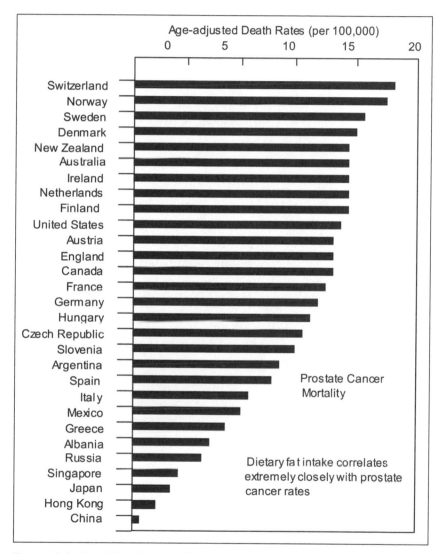

Figure 2.1. Prostate Cancer Mortality Rates. This figure compares the prostate cancer-related death rates per 100,000 people in twenty-nine countries. Note that the people of China, who traditionally eat a very low-fat diet, have the lowest number of prostate-related deaths.

Eat temperate nuts like almonds, walnuts, pine nuts, and pecans, rather than tropical ones like cashews and Brazil nuts (though people native to tropical areas certainly can eat these). There is no one botanical category of "tree nuts," as every one is completely different in species and unrelated to any others. *The concept of "tree nut allergies" is completely ridiculous.*

THE PROOF IS IN YOUR FAT

The American Health Foundation in Valhalla, New York, has done a fine job of showing how a low-fat, high-fiber diet slows the development of prostate cancer. Native South African black men have extremely low prostate disease rates on their traditional diets. When fed a typical American high-fat diet, their testosterone levels fell, their estrogen levels rose (and thus, their testosterone-to-estrogen ratio worsened), and they got more prostate disease (*Bulletin of the New York Academy of Medicine* v 56, 1980 and *Cancer Research* v 42, 1982).

Again, the American Health Foundation carried out an in-depth review of the scientific studies to show that omega-6 fatty acids stimulate prostate cancer growth, while omega-3 fatty acids (like flax oil) inhibit it (*Journal of the National Cancer Institute* v 85, 1993). The problem is that the omega-3s are rare in foods, while omega-6s are all too common. Red meat contains arachidonic acid and linoleic acid, which are generally nonexistent in plant foods. These are considered to be the most dangerous and inflammatory fatty acids known.

A third study there (*Lipids* v 27, 1992) stated, "International comparisons suggest a relationship between prostate cancer incidence and dietary fat, an inference supported by migration studies. N-6 [or omega-6] fatty acids stimulate and N-3 [omega-3] fatty acids inhibit human prostate cells." They presented overwhelming clinical studies to support these findings. Their charts were inarguable proof.

Doctors at Sina Hospital in Tehran (*Nutrition and Cancer* v 63, 2011) said total fat consumption increases prostate cancer risk. The

University of Chicago (*Journal of Urology* v 177, 2007) explained Jamaica has the highest prostate cancer rate in the entire world. They have a very high fat diet and eat far too much linoleic (omega-6) fatty acids. "Our findings support the association of dietary fatty acids and prostate cancer." At Harvard (*JNCI* v 85, 1993) they made it very clear, "Total fat consumption was directly related to risk of advanced prostate cancer, primarily to animal fat."

At the University of Laval (*Journal of Urology* v 159, 1998) they found total fat, saturated fat, monosaturated fat, polyunsaturated fat, linoleic acid, total vegetable fat, and total animal fat all were strongly correlated with advanced prostate cancer. At the International Cancer Research in London (*British Journal of Nutrition* v103, 2010), it was concluded, "There was a positive association between prostate cancer risk and dietary intake of total fat and fat subtypes."

Again, at Harvard (*Cancer Causes and Controls* v 26, 2015), they studied men with prostate cancer as to their mortality: "Men who obtained 5 percent more of their daily calorics from saturated fat had a 1.8 fold increased risk of mortality." A stunning review was done at the University of Wales (*British Journal of Urology* v 77, 1996), which found that "the Western Diet is characterized by a high content of animal fat, animal protein, low fibre, and refined carbohydrates." Epidemiological studies repeatedly show this regiment to be strongly correlated with all types of prostate disease. At the New Orleans Charity Hospital (*Prostate Cancer, Prostate Diseases* v 20, 2017) 1,854 men with PC were studied. High total fat- adjusted saturated fat intake was associated with increased prostate cancer aggressiveness. At five hospitals in Jinan, China, (*Zhonghua Fangzhi* v 14, 2007) it was discovered, "The tests found there is a dose response between prostate cancer and total energy, total fat, saturated fats, and animal fat."

CONCLUSION

We have conclusively shown that fat intake, especially from animal fat, is the biggest factor in prostate disease. The more fats you eat, especially saturated fats, the more chance you have of getting prostate cancer, BPH, and prostatitis. Would you rather eat meat, poultry, eggs, and dairy products, and die a painful, lingering, premature death? Or would you rather change your diet and live a healthier, happier, longer life? Eating fat raises your estradiol and estrone levels, causes all manner of illness, and makes you obese. This is the main reason American and European men over the age of fifty have higher estrogen levels than women of the same age! That's right, Western men over fifty generally have more estrogen (estradiol and estrone) in their blood than their wives do after menopause! This is frightening!

Fat intake also increases the levels of harmful "free radicals" in our bodies. Free radicals are molecules with unpaired electrons. They damage our health by attacking healthy cells in an attempt to balance the electrical charge they carry. Referred to as "oxidative damage," this effect not only harms our metabolism, but makes for a poor quality of life and causes early mortality. Oxidative damage is a major factor in aging. By making better food choices, you can lower the amount of free radicals in your body and live a longer, healthier life.

The ideal diet contains only 10 percent fat calories from vegetables (or even seafood). The maximum is 20 percent fat calories from vegetables. Eating any more fat than this will simply not benefit you. You must eat less than one-fifth of your calories as fats and oils, and no more than that. Lowering fat intake from 40 percent fat calories to, say, 25 percent just won't do anything at all. *To benefit from a low-fat diet, you must eat less than 20 percent fat calories, preferably about 10 percent.* Pseudoscientific "studies" will lower fat calorie intake to around 30 percent, and then claim there were no benefits found—no wonder! Achieving good health is not difficult to do when you simply make better food choices. Taking meat, poultry, eggs, and dairy out of your daily fare will basically solve the problem.

3. Supplements

Always remember that continually making better food choices is the most important thing we can do for our health. *Natural health is about diet and lifestyle.* Lifestyle factors include supplements, exercise, stress, smoking, alcohol intake, prescription and recreational drug use, fasting, and bad habits like caffeine. Supplements are important, but very secondary to diet. You receive far more health benefits with both proper diet *and* supplements than with diet alone.

All of the supplements discussed in this chapter are natural, safe, and inexpensive. They all have numerous published clinical studies behind them that show their value to prostate health, and to health in general. This chapter is not going to use extensive references, however. Please just realize that all of these supplements have been proven effective after four decades of published human clinical research.

Some supplements are measured in international units (IU), while others in milligrams (mg), or micrograms (mcg). International units measure the strength or potency of a substance, while milligrams and micrograms measure its weight.

SUPPLEMENTS FOR YOUR TOTAL HEALTH

Our diets lack the proper nutrients, and proven supplements can solve that. There are so many supplements on the market, it is difficult to determine which ones really work. The following list of supplements is for your overall health.

BETA-CAROTENE

Beta-carotene is a powerful, proven, and well-known antioxidant. A study published in *Cancer Research* showed that the intake of beta-carotene had a strong correlation with reduced prostate cancer in Japanese men. Many other studies have shown similar results. Supplementing your diet with beta-carotene is better than taking vitamin A because beta-carotene is a precursor to vitamin A, so you won't overload your body, even with higher doses.

Dosage

Beta-carotene is an important antioxidant with many health benefits, so take 10,000 IU daily. Most companies offer 25,000 IU, but this is simply too much. More is not better.

BETA-SITOSTEROL

Sterols are plant alcohols that occur in every vegetable you eat. Clinical studies over the last forty years have shown that beta-sitosterol is the most important supplement for good prostate (and cholesterol) health. A more accurate term is "mixed sterols." The studies on sterols are listed in Chapter 5.

It's very important you understand that herbal products such as saw palmetto, pygeum, nettles, etc., contain almost no (generally one-thirtieth of one percent) mixed sterols, even though they are the active ingredients. These products are of no value. Analytical testing has shown that there are simply no biologically significant amounts of sterols—even in the most expensive extracts. To prove this to yourself, just read the label;

you will not find beta-sitosterol or mixed sterols listed. There are no other active ingredients! There are also no human tests that suggest these products are actually effective.

Dosage

Take 300 mg to 600 mg of mixed sterols a day. Make sure the label says at least 300 mg of mixed plant sterols.

COENZYME Q10

Coenzyme Q10, or CoQ10, is a powerful enzyme in our bodies, but our CoQ10 levels fall as we age. Studies have shown that CoQ10 helps prevent and cure various forms of cancer, as well as other diseases. At Nagoya University in Japan, scientists found that when CoQ10 was added to cells taken from BPH patients, it had a very beneficial effect on their metabolism. CoQ10 has amazing health benefits for our heart, brain, kidneys, liver, and other organs. Everyone over forty should take this supplement.

Dosage

You must take at least 100 mg of CoQ10 daily. If you are sickly, or have cancer, take 200 mg daily for one year. Be sure to take at least 100 mg a day of real Japanese ubiquinone (CoQ10), even though many brands offer less than 100 mg. The price of real Japanese CoQ10 is as low as twenty dollars for sixty capsules. Do *not* take ubiquinol, as it is unstable and has no shelf life. The label *must* say Japanese ubiquinone. Take this with your food or flax oil.

FLAXSEED OIL

Flaxseed oil is very good for prostate health, and the best known source of omega-3 fatty acids. Consuming 1,000 to 2,000 mg (1/2 teaspoon) of omega-3 fatty acids daily is good for people of all ages. "The Health Professionals Follow-up Study" analyzed the diets of 51,529 men. Their research showed that omega-6 fatty acids were positively associated with prostate cancer rates. Omega-3 fatty acids, on the other hand, were associated with prostate health.

In Beijing, researchers at Peking Medical College gave men flax extract for four months. This dramatically increased their urine flow, as well as their International Prostate Symptom Score, or IPSS. This is based on a questionnaire made up of various important diagnostic factors, and is the most accepted diagnostic measurement of prostate health. A study involving prostate cancer patients was done at Duke University. Men given a flax supplement slowed down their cancer growth in only thirty-four days. When self-appointed Internet authorities tell you that flax oil is bad for prostate health, now you'll know they walk in darkness. The more research done on omega-3s and flaxseed oil, the more health benefits are revealed.

Flaxseed is the best source of omega-3 fatty acids. Flax oil supplements are preferable to fish liver or krill oil supplements for many reasons. Flax has more omega-3s, and is less subject to rancidity. Flax contains linolenic acid, while fish contains DHA and EPA. The many studies on omega-3 fatty acids that used fish liver oils are equally applicable to flax oil. There are many good reasons to take flax daily, especially for cardiovascular health.

Dosage

Just 1,000 mg a day of flax oil is very beneficial and only nine calories. When you buy flax oil, make sure it has been refrigerated, and keep it refrigerated to prevent oxidation.

GLUTATHIONE

Glutathione is one of our four basic antioxidant enzymes, and it is a critical part of our immune system. Glutathione levels are important for prostate health, but blood and tissue glutathione levels typically fall as people age. Taking glutathione alone is expensive, as well as ineffective. Fortunately, you can take an inexpensive 600 mg capsule of N-acetyl cysteine, or NAC, to enhance your glutathione levels very effectively and safely. In the last few years, there has been quite a bit of good research published on the value of NAC supplements. By maintaining a youthful glutathione level, you will gain many health benefits; in particular, boosting your glutathione levels will improve your immune system, so you can better resist disease.

Dosage

Take 600 mg of NAC daily. NAC is widely available, so buy any good brand.

MINERALS

Minerals are essential for prostate health, and we are woefully mineral deficient. No matter how well you eat, you just aren't going to get all the minerals you need because our farm and crop soils are in such poor conditions and lacking in so many elements. Minerals work synergistically, so you need all of them to be healthy. We have only begun to study the importance of minerals on prostate function, but it is already clear that you will never have good prostate health as long as you are mineral deficient.

Find a mineral supplement that contains the required amounts of all the known elements our bodies need. We get enough sodium, potassium, sulfur, and phosphorous in our diets already. This includes boron, calcium, chromium, cobalt, copper, iodine, iron, magnesium, manganese, molybdenum, nickel, selenium, silicon, strontium, tin, vanadium, and zinc. The two most important minerals for prostate health are selenium and zinc. However, the point is to get all the minerals you need, and not just the two most important.

The multivitamin and mineral supplements you see generally have only about ten of these elements. Look for a mineral-only supplement that contains at least these seventeen vital minerals in the amounts you need. Try searching the Internet for "mineral supplements." Avoid colloidal minerals and ionic minerals, as these do not contain any biologically significant mineral amounts. *Read the label* to see which minerals are included, and in what amounts.

In 2016, the FDA irrationally banned any germanium, cesium, or gallium in vitamin supplements. It is important to realize that we need all of the known minerals. In the future, science will probably show that we need other minerals such as barium, rubidium, europium, neodymium, praseodymium, thulium, lithium, samarium, tungsten, lanthanum, and yttrium. Barium is a regular trace element and we take in about 1,000 mcg daily. Rubidium is also a regular trace element and we take in about 1,000 mcg of that as well. There are definitely ultra-trace elements that will eventually prove to be vital. These include those minerals listed above as well as several others, which will be discussed further in Chapter 4.

Dosage

To learn the optimal daily intake for each of these vital minerals, refer to Table 3.1 on page 38. This table provides you with the appropriate doses of twenty minerals. In the following chapter, each mineral is discussed in detail, so you can learn the specific benefits of these essential nutrients.

QUERCETIN

Quercetin is a potent and proven plant-derived antioxidant, but it is not yet well known. You will hear more about this effective supplement. Studies in the *Journal of Steroid Biochemistry, Urology*, and the Japanese journal *Daizu Tanpakushitsu Kenkyukai Kaishi* show that quercetin can help promote prostate health. A new study at the Mayo Clinic, published in *Carcinogenesis*, suggests that quercetin may have real value in fighting against prostate cancer. Quercetin is a beneficial supplement for many other reasons besides being an excellent antioxidant. It isn't found in very high amounts, if at all, in many common foods, though.

Dosage

A daily dosage of 100 mg of any brand is good, as a normal diet only provides about 10 mg (mostly from apples and onions). Don't take more than this. More is not better.

SOY ISOFLAVONES

Soy isoflavones have a lot of published, clinical, human research proving their health benefits. Studies have shown that these isoflavones support prostate health. The main components in soy that we are concerned with are genistein and daidzein (and equol). These are flavones (plant pigments), and unrelated to hormones or prohormones (precursors to hormones). *Genistein and daidzein are not "phytoestrogens."* There is no estrogen, or any other hormone-testosterone, progesterone, dehydroepiandrosterone (DHEA), melatonin, etc., in plants. Soy does not have estrogenic effects. *There is no such thing as a phytoestrogen!*

Studies on soy benefits for prostate health have been published in journals such as *Prostate, Anti-Cancer Research, Journal of Endocrinology, Nutrition and Cancer, Journal of Steroid Biochemistry, Cancer Epidemiology, Biomarkers & Prevention, American Journal of Clinical Nutrition, Cancer Letters, International Journal of Oncology,* and many others. The proof here is overwhelming. You may see Internet sites warning against the "dangers" of soy, but this is simply propaganda from the dairy and meat industries (especially the Weston Price Foundation and American Dairy Association).

Dosage

A good brand of soy isoflavones will list the amount of genistein and daidzein on the label. Take a total of 40 mg daily. Soy foods, especially refined foods such as tofu, generally are an impractical source of isoflavones. Soy isoflavone supplements are a much more practical and realistic means of isoflavone intake. Using soy milk regularly is another.

VITAMIN D

Vitamin D deficiency is a worldwide epidemic. Vitamin D does not occur in our food in any meaningful amount. Vitamin D3, the most important "vitamin" for your prostate, is really a hormone that is produced in our bodies when we are exposed to sunlight.

Most of the research on vitamin D and the prostate has been done only in the last fifteen years. There are hundreds of clinical studies demonstrating the importance of vitamin D in prostate function. These include studies in such journals as *Cancer Research, Anticancer Research, Prostate, Clinical Cancer Research, Cancer Letters, Surgical Forum,* and other respected international publications. One study at Stanford University, which treated men with prostate cancer with no other therapy than vitamin D supplements, had very impressive results.

Dosage

Take 800 IU of vitamin D a day (unless you're out in the sun often); this is a safe amount, especially in wintertime when we get little exposure to the sun. Vitamin D3 is fat-soluble, so don't listen to "experts" who tell you to take more than this. Do not take more than 1,200 IU, and don't take it if you are regularly exposed to sunlight. Continue taking your usual vitamins as normal.

VITAMIN E

Vitamin E is a very beneficial nutrient, especially for our cardiovascular health. Our American diets are generally very deficient in vitamin E. Whole grains are the best source of vitamin E, but most of us eat only one percent whole grains, instead of 50 percent. This is the second-most important vitamin for your prostate. There are countless published studies from around the world that show the value of vitamin E supplementation for prostate health, and for health in general. Every year more studies are published. Vitamin E is a basic and proven supplement for people of all ages, but many other vitamins are also essential to our health. The inset on page 38 provides more information on vitamins.

Dosage

Your daily vitamin pill will contain the Reference Daily Intake (RDI) of vitamin E, but that's only 30 IU. Supplement your diet with 200 IU daily of mixed natural tocopherols, and note that this is seven times the RDI. Or take a 400 IU capsule every other day. Be careful not to take too much, because overdoses will thin your blood. And don't use the cheap brands that contain only d-alpha tocopherol. Take mixed tocopherols.

Vitamins are important. There are only thirteen vitamins, and there is an RDI set for each. Be especially careful when selecting vitamin B and vitamin C supplements. Be sure to find a multivitamin with one mg of methylcobalamin instead of regular cobalamin vitamin B12 (cobalamin). Vitamin B12 is just not orally absorbed, but methylcobalamin is.

We only need about 60 mg a day of vitamin C, and that is supplied in our daily food. Taking more than 250 mg a day of vitamin C is harmful and will, over time, acidify your blood and make you sick. Your blood is naturally alkaline, having a pH level of 7.4. Megadoses of any nutrient unbalance the body's metabolism. *Do not take more than 250 mg of vitamin C a day.* For all other vitamins, simply take the recommended daily intake.

ACIDOPHILUS

Acidophilus, and other probiotics, show no specific benefit for prostate health per se, but are important to add to your supplements list. Our bodies work as a holistic system, and our digestion is obviously vital to our total health. *Good health begins with our digestion.* Our digestive tracts are generally in terrible shape from overeating, and from eating the wrong foods. Consuming whole, healthy foods, eating lower calorie foods, fasting one day a week, and taking a good brand of acidophilus daily can dramatically improve your digestive system.

Dosage

A good brand of acidophilus should state that every capsule has at least six billion live multi-strain organisms and eight different strains at the time of manufacture. Do not be misled by "per gram" counts, rather than per capsule. Buy it, and keep it refrigerated. If you can find stronger brands with more strains, that is even better.

FRUCTO-OLIGOSACCHARIDES

Fructo-oligosaccharides (FOS), otherwise known as inulin, works well with glutamine (another important supplement discussed in this chapter) and acidophilus. FOS is an indigestible saccharide that is extracted from various plants (such as chicory). It feeds the good Lacto and Bifido bacteria in our intestines. FOS is called a "prebiotic" and works synergistically with probiotics. The health benefits of FOS have been known for a long time, but it is only recently that the intestinal health benefits have been discovered. Good human studies have been published on this.

Dosage

Take 750 to 1,500 mg of FOS daily. Remember that 90 percent of our immunity comes from our digestive system. Our digestive system is the very center of our health.

BETA GLUCAN

Beta glucan is the most potent immune system-enhancing supplement known to science. It has been studied for its power against tumors and cancer. It doesn't matter whether beta glucan comes from yeast and mushrooms (1,3/1,6 configuration) or oats and barley (1,3/1,4 configuration). All 1,3 configurations of true beta glucan polysaccharides have the same potency.

Beta glucan has proven power to stimulate our immune system. It has an amazing ability to fight infections and ward off illnesses. The power of beta glucan has been known for over thirty years now. This is definitely a supplement people of all ages need to take. Yet, only in the last decade have advances in technology allowed us to extract it easily and inexpensively. Currently, yeast is the least expensive source of beta glucan. Read my booklet *What Is Beta Glucan?*

Dosage

Economical 400 mg supplements are available for about ten dollars for sixty capsules. Still, there is a lot of advertising misinformation about beta glucan, especially on the Internet. Be careful when selecting the right brand for you. Don't listen to ads claiming special configurations and other such nonsense. It doesn't matter whether it is derived from oats, barley, mushrooms, or yeast. Look for the best deal on a reliable product.

DI-INDOLYL METHANE

Di-indolyl methane (DIM) is the direct metabolite of indole-3-carbinol, or I3C. There are excellent studies on both DIM and I3C that show they lower serum estrogen levels, and have anticancer effects. These studies have been published in *Cancer Research, Journal of the National Cancer Association, Anticancer Research, Annals of the New York Academy of Sciences,* and other major journals. I3C is found in cruciferous vegetables (cabbage, broccoli, Brussels sprouts, and cauliflower), but it is less expensive, and more practical, to take 200 mg a day of DIM rather than 400 mg a day of I3C. DIM is a much better bargain, and twice as powerful.

High estrogen levels in our bodies cause many problems as we age. Taking DIM is an excellent way to reduce estrogen levels and improve estrogen metabolism. If your levels of free estradiol and estrone test are low to normal, you do not need to take this. Maintaining a low-fat diet and exercising can keep estrogen levels low. Do not buy overpriced DIM with a "special delivery system." Just take DIM with your meals or flax oil, as it is fat soluble.

Dosage

Taking 200 mg of DIM a day can improve your estrogen metabolism and lower powerful estradiol and estrone levels. This is synergistic with flax or fish oil.

GLUCOSAMINE

Glucosamine is a basic supplement for bone and joint health. 95 percent of Americans over the age of sixty-five have some form of arthritis. Glucosamine is an important addition to your diet. There is good science behind glucosamine if it is used properly. Glucosamine works very well with cofactors such as minerals, flax oil, soy isoflavones, and vitamin D. Moreover, glucosamine needs hormones such as testosterone, DHEA, estriol (in women), and progesterone.

Dosage

Take 500 to 1,000 mg of glucosamine a day. Remember that chondroitin (a supplement derived from animal cartilage) is useless, despite its popularity. The molecule is too large to pass through the digestive walls and into the blood. Always remember that glucosamine needs cofactors to be effective.

L-GLUTAMINE

Glutamine is an amino acid with many health benefits, especially in strengthening digestive and intestinal function. Several good studies have shown how glutamine improves our intestinal health, and it works well in concert with acidophilus and FOS. Good digestion is central to good health. Our digestion is generally weak from lifelong dietary abuse, but glutamine, along with acidophilus and FOS, improves digestion.

Dosage

You should take at least 1,000 mg to 2,000 mg (four 500 mg tablets) of L-glutamine a day (two tablets in the A.M. and two in the

P.M.). You can also buy bulk glutamine powder, and take one tablespoon (about 2.5 grams) a day. It is tasteless, and can easily be added to your food, or dissolved in soy milk.

LIPOIC ACID

Lipoic acid levels in our bodies fall as we age, and unfortunately, this supplement is not found in our food. There are a lot of excellent scientific studies that show lipoic acid is good for brain metabolism, coronary heart health, and blood sugar metabolism. Insulin resistance, high blood sugar, high insulin, metabolic syndrome, and diabetes are epidemics in Western society now. One in three American children will grow up diabetic—due mainly to our insane intake of 160 pounds of various sugars every year.

Your blood sugar should be 85 mg/dL (milligrams per deciliter) or less, and lipoic acid can help you achieve healthy blood sugar levels. Supplementing your diet with lipoic acid is very important for anyone over the age of forty, or anyone with a blood sugar level over 85 mg/dL.

Dosage

You should take 400 mg of regular R,S-lipoic acid a day in order to maintain normal blood sugar levels. Take 400 mg and no less. Do not take R-only lipoic acid because it's expensive, and there are no human tests that even suggest this form is actually more effective. Nearly all of the clinical studies on lipoic acid have used the regular mixed R,S-isomer.

PHOSPHATIDYL SERINE

Phosphatidyl serine (PS) is very important for brain function, memory, and preventing Alzheimer's disease and senility. PS is found mostly in our brains and nervous system, and clinical studies on PS have shown that it can help prevent the loss of our mental faculties as we age. This is now extracted from soybeans.

Dosage

PS is a very effective supplement, but works best with other brain healthy nutrients. Take 100 mg of PS a day, and use this with pregnenolone. Only in the last few years has PS become available to us inexpensively from soybeans. Lecithin, or phosphatidylcholine, is also a very good time-proven supplement, especially for heart and artery health. Take 1,200 mg of lecithin a day if you want to add another proven supplement.

SUPPLEMENTS FOR TEMPORARY USE

There are some good exogenous, temporary supplements you can take if you like. *Exogenous* supplements are not found in your body, or in your daily food. After about six months, most of the exogenous supplements listed below lose their effect. Only take them temporarily. These simply don't work for everyone.

ALOE VERA

Aloe vera has been known for centuries for its healing power both inside and out. Daily supplements for six months will help strengthen your digestive system. It can even help heal the lining of your stomach and the walls of your intestines. Aloe is a time-proven herbal remedy that works well with acidophilus, FOS, and glutamine.

Dosage

Take two 100 mg capsules of a 200:1 aloe vera extract a day for up to six months. Stop if you get a laxative effect.

CURCUMIN

Curcumin is an extract from the culinary herb turmeric, and it is a clinically proven powerful anti-inflammatory. A study on prostate cancer at the Comprehensive Cancer Center in New York City showed that curcumin "has the potential to prevent the progression of [prostate] cancer . . ." Additional studies on curcumin and cancer have been in *Molecular Urology, FEBS Letters, Molecular Medicine,* and other journals.

Dosage

Take 500 mg of curcumin daily for up to six months.

ELLAGIC ACID

Ellagic acid has shown good anticancer activity in many studies; it can help prevent cancer, stop the growth of tumors, and even kill cancer cells. It is commonly found in black walnut hulls, as well as some fruits and other nuts in smaller amounts. Ellagic acid has been known to herbalists for years. As research continues, you will hear more about its benefits.

Dosage

Unfortunately, most available brands are overpriced, and their labels are very misleading. Often they list the amount of extract, but not the actual amount of actual ellagic acid. Find a brand with a label that states 200 mg, or more, of actual ellagic acid. Make sure you buy an extract that clearly and honestly states the potency *per capsule,* not "per dose." Take at least 200 mg of ellagic acid a day for up to six months.

FRUIT PECTIN

Fruit pectin, as part of a total program of diet and supplements, has been shown to help prevent prostate cancer, prostatitis, and BPH. Studies have shown that fruit pectin supplements effectively lower cholesterol and improve digestion. It even has general anticancer properties, so it can prevent and cure various other cancers, as well as prostate cancer.

Dosage

Take 3 g or more a day, in caplets or as powder (it's tasteless) in fruit juice for up to six months. Do not waste your money on expensive "modified" pectin. You don't need to modify pectin. Just buy the plain, inexpensive, regular kind, like grapefruit or apple pectin. Regular fruit pectin is soluble, bioavailable, and very beneficial in many ways (besides lowering cholesterol levels).

GREEN TEA EXTRACT

Hundreds of published clinical studies on both animals and humans have shown that green tea extract helps alleviate prostate disease. Green tea contains valuable and powerful antioxidants like polyphenols and cathechins. This is the same tea you see everywhere, before fermenting changes its color to black.

Dosage

Taking green tea extract supplements is more practical than trying to drink green tea every day. Yes, many Japanese drink green tea daily, but it is caffeinated. Many inexpensive brands of 95 percent decaffeinated green tea extract are available. Take two 300 mg capsules of 95 percent decaffeinated extract a day. Again, because green tea extract is exogenous, you only need to take it for up to six months.

MILK THISTLE

Milk thistle has many potential health benefits, particularly for the prostate. Milk thistle is a well-known and time-proven herb because of its powerful active ingredient, silymarin. Studies in many international journals such as *Cancer Letters* and *Cancer Research* have shown that taking milk thistle has very promising effects on our prostate health. This is a very important herb for liver health as well. Use this with TMG for liver rejuvenation.

Dosage

Two capsules a day of a good milk thistle extract will give you about 200 mg of silymarin. After about six months you can stop using milk thistle, as all exogenous herbs lose their effect after that time. This goes very well with TMG.

SODIUM ALGINATE

Sodium alginate is a seaweed extract that has many proven health benefits. The most dramatic benefit of sodium alginate is that it can remove toxic heavy metals from our blood. When sodium alginate binds to heavy metals (such as mercury, lead, and cadmium) in our blood, these substances are then safely excreted from our bodies through our feces.

Dosage

Take 3 g of sodium alginate a day for up to six months. Weekly fasting also helps to remove heavy metals and other toxins. You can repeat this every day, for five years.

TRIMETHYLGLYCINE

Trimethylglycine (TMG), also known as betaine, is an amino acid found in our food. Studies have shown that it has powerful rejuvenating and detoxifying effects on our livers. In fact, TMG is the best liver rejuvenator known to science. Use this with milk thistle.

Dosage

Take 3 g of TMG a day for up to six months. You can also take one g a day permanently to help maintain lower homocysteine levels. (High homocysteine levels are an important diagnostic marker of heart disease.) You can repeat this liver cleanse every, say, five years, but only if you have a problem with your liver as diagnosed by the ALT/SGOT and AST/SGPT blood levels.

SUPPLEMENTS TO AVOID

Over twenty years of research, it has become obvious that most of those "wonder supplements" so heavily promoted by the natural health industry simply have no scientific evidence behind them. Such products include:

- acai berries
- Active hexose correlated compound (AHCC)
- artemisia (wormwood)
- astaxanthin
- bee products (pollen, jelly, propolis, etc.)
- bilberry
- Cat's claw (uña de gato)
- cetyl myristoleate (CMO)
- chondroitin
- chorella
- chrysin
- citrus pectin
- Conjugated Linoleic Acid (CLA)
- colloidal minerals
- colloidal silver
- colon cleansers
- colostrum
- coral calcium
- deer antler velvet
- dimethylaminoetha-nol (DMAE)
- goji berries
- "greens"
- Gymnema sylvestre
- HGH secretagogues
- homeopathic remediesarginine
- hoodia cactus
- hyaluronic acid
- 5-hydroxytryptamine (5-HTP)
- ionic minerals
- maca root
- mangosteen products
- MGN-3
- MSM
- muira puama
- nattokinase
- oral chelation
- oral S.O.D.
- pomegranate products
- policosanol
- Pyrroquinoline quinone (PQQ)
- Pygeum africanum
- red rice yeast
- resveratrol
- saw palmetto
- sexual rejuvenation formulas
- shark cartilage
- spirulina

- suma
- Tongkat ali
- Tribulus terrestis
- ubiquinol
- whey protein

Lycopene, for example, simply has no good published science behind it. Actual blood serum studies prove that there is no correlation between lycopene levels and prostate health (*Journal of the National Cancer Institute* v 82, 1990 and *Cancer Epidemiology Biomarkers Preview* v 6, 1997). At Johns Hopkins University (*Prostate* v 47, 2001), the blood of 25,802 men was analyzed for nutrients and matched with their medical records. No relation was found with lycopene content. At the Cancer Research Center in Honolulu (*Igaku No Ayumi* v 103, 1977), the blood of 6,850 men was analyzed for nutrients, and no relation with serum lycopene levels was found. In fact, tomatoes must be cooked in oil in order for their lycopene to be absorbable. It is clear that actual blood studies on men show no relation at all between serum lycopene levels and prostate health. Plasma lycopene levels are worthless.

AN OVERVIEW OF IMPORTANT DAILY SUPPLEMENTS

The table below lists the most important supplements you should take on a permanent basis in order to improve the health of your prostate and your health in general. Beside the name of each supplement, you'll find the optimal daily intake, which is not necessarily the same as the reference daily intake (RDI) established by the Food and Drug Administration (FDA).

Note, for example, that the RDI for vitamin E is only 30 IU, but the optimal daily intake is 200 IU. Vitamin E is very important for prostate health, but most of us don't get enough vitamin E through our normal diets.

TABLE 3.1. PERMANENT DAILY SUPPLEMENTS

Supplements	Optimal Daily Intake	Considerations
VITAMINS		
Vitamin B1 (Thiamine)	1.5 mg	
Vitamin B2 (Riboflavin)	1.75 mg	
Vitamin B3 (Niacin)	20 mg	
Vitamin B6	2 mg	
Vitamin B12	2 mg	As methyl cobalamin
Vitamin C	60 mg	Do not take more than 250 mg in one day.
Vitamin D	800 IU	Do not take more than 1,200 IU a day.
Vitamin E	200 IU of mixed natural tocopherols	Or take 400 IU every other day.
Vitamin K	80 mcg	
Biotin	300 mcg	
Folate (Folic Acid)	400 mcg	
Pantothenic Acid	10 mg	
MINERALS		
Boron	3 mg	
Calcium	250 mg	Some suggest taking 1,000 mg of calcium a day, but only dairy intake will give you this much calcium, and it is better to avoid eating dairy.
Cesium	100 mcg	Now banned by the FDA
Chromium	120 mcg	
Cobalt	25 mcg	
Copper	2 mg	
Gallium	100 mcg	Now banned by the FDA

Supplements	Optimal Daily Intake	Considerations
Germanium	100 mcg	Now banned by the FDA
Iodine	150 mcg	
Iron	10 mg for men, 18 mg for women	
Magnesium	400 mg	
Manganese	2 mg	
Molybdenum	75 mcg	
Nickel	100 mcg	
Selenium	70 mcg	
Silicon	10 mg	
Strontium	one mg	
Tin	100 mcg	Limited to 30 mcg by the FDA
Vanadium	one mg (1,000 mcg)	
Zinc	15 mg	
OTHER NUTRIENTS		
Acidophilus	6 billion live multi-strain organism capsules or more	Buy and keep refrigerated. Take once or twice daily.
Beta-carotene	10,000 IU	25,000 IU is an overdose
Beta Glucan	400 mg or more	
Beta-sitosterol Complex	300 to 600 mg	
Coenzyme Q10	100 mg	Take with food, or flax oil as Coenzyme Q10 is oil-soluble.
Di-indolyl Methane (DIM)	200 mg	Take with food, or flax oil as DIM is oil-soluble.
Flaxseed Oil	1,000 to 2,000 mg	Buy and keep refrigerated. Take once or twice daily.
Fructo-oligosaccharides (FOS)	750 to 1,500 mg	

Supplements	Optimal Daily Intake	Considerations
Glucosamine	500 to 1,000 mg	Needs co-factors
L-glutamine	1,000 to 2,000 mg	Take half in the A.M. and half in the P.M.
Lipoic Acid	400 mg	
N-acetyl Cysteine (Glutathione)	600 mg	
Phosphatidyl Serine (PS)	100 mg	
Quercetin	100 mg	
Soy Isoflavones	40 mg of daidzein and genistein	If you drink soy milk regularly, you probably don't need this.

Animal proteins such as acetyl-L-carnitine (or any form of carnitine) and L-carnosine are no longer recommended. Animal proteins, per se, have been shown to promote disease, along with the saturated fat and cholesterol content of meat, poultry, eggs, and dairy products.

CONCLUSION

There are forty-seven permanent supplements recommended in this chapter for men over forty. These are the very same supplements recommended for women, by the way. You should take these supplements in addition to any hormones you need. Use as many supplements listed in Table 3.1 as you possibly can, as they have many overall health benefits.

Poor health in general contributes to your prostate condition. Don't choose surgery, radiation, or dangerous prescription drugs because you may end up wearing diapers, losing your sexual ability, or dying a tortuous, premature death. An *ounce of prevention is worth ten pounds of cure.* These natural, proven products will help both prevent and cure your health problems. Supplements are only one of the *Seven Steps to Natural Health* (see page 119).

4. The Minerals You Need

Studies have shown us how important minerals are to prostate metabolism and to health in general. Good mineral nutrition helps us live longer, healthier lives. Though zinc, selenium, and chromium have gotten the most attention, many minerals are vital to our nutrition. *Every disease or medical condition is due in part to mineral deficiency.* We are all mineral deficient, no matter how well we eat or where we live. We need all the known minerals for human nutrition, not just some of them.

Minerals, like hormones, work together as a team. There are at least twenty-four known elements needed for human nutrition. Of those twenty-four, we get enough phosphorous, potassium, sodium, and sulfur in our food, so we do not need to supplement these minerals. The best, most expensive mineral supplements available only have about ten different elements. Few supplements in the world provide all of the known minerals we need in the necessary servings. Just Google "mineral supplements" to find one that does. A detailed list of these twenty minerals, along with the recommended dosage of each, follows.

BORON

Boron is probably the most deficient mineral in your diet. Americans probably only ingest one mg of boron a day, but actually need three times this amount. You would think all mineral supplements would contain a mere 3 mg of this inexpensive and vital element, but many do not. This is just another case of megacorporations and manufacturers that have huge advertising budgets, but no research departments. It wasn't until 1990 that boron was officially considered an essential part of your diet! The research is overwhelming here. Our soils and food are very lacking in boron. Boron deficiency is all too common, so be sure your supplement has at least 3 mg per dose.

Dosage

There is no official recommended daily intake (RDI) for boron, but 3 mg is commonly suggested. Citrates or common boric acid are excellent sources of boron.

CALCIUM

Calcium, in any significant quantity, is only found in dairy foods. You should not eat dairy foods. The RDI of 1,000 mg is completely scientifically unfounded. Asians, for example, generally only take in about 250 mg of calcium a day, and they tend to have far fewer bone and joint problems than we Americans do.

Dosage

Take 250 mg of calcium a day. Be sure to take flax oil, minerals, and vitamin D as well, because calcium needs cofactors in order for it to be absorbed. Do not take more than this.

CESIUM

Cesium is an important ultra-trace mineral, so you only need 100 mcg a day; do not take more than this. Human blood, common food, and soil studies have proven how vital cesium is for our health, and yet you will never find it in mineral supplements. Internationally published studies have also shown the importance of cesium in our soil, our food, and our blood. Cesium is vital for human health, and soon science must admit this fact and set an RDI for cesium. Instead, the FDA banned cesium in supplements in 2016.

Dosage

Because cesium is an ultra-trace mineral, you only need to take 100 mcg a day. Regular salts, especially chloride, can provide you with enough cesium.

CHROMIUM

Only recently has chromium been given an RDI of 120 mcg. Chromium is often deficient in our diet because we tend to eat refined grains instead of whole grains. Science has proven that chromium is critical for proper prostate metabolism. Chromium deficiency is one of the many reasons prostate disease is such an epidemic.

Dosage

The RDI for chromium is 120 mcg. Never take more than 400 mcg a day, and do not listen to advertisements that claim their form of chromium is the "only effective one." Regular chelates (nonmetal ions that bond to a metal ion for better absorbability) are the best source of chromium. Simply look for a bottle labeled "chromium chelate."

COBALT

Even though it is the basic building block for vitamin B-12, cobalt is almost never found in mineral supplements. Food and blood studies have proven the importance of cobalt for our health. Our bodies are supposed to synthesize our own vitamin B-12, but that process cannot occur without cobalt in our blood.

Sufficient amounts of vitamin B-12 are just not found in foods, and B-12 is ineffective when taken orally. Just 25 mcg of cobalt is enough to help the body produce adequate amounts of vitamin B-12. To help ensure healthy B-12 levels, take one mcg of methylcobalamin in addition to cobalt. Methylcobalamin is a type of B-12 that is very absorbable.

Dosage

In order to insure that your body can produce at least 3 mcg of vitamin B-12 a day, you should take 25 mcg of cobalt.

COPPER

Copper has an RDI of only 2 mg. Still, Americans probably only consume about half this amount. Whole grains and beans are the best source of copper, but most of us don't eat enough of these foods. Your body only contains about 150 mg of this vital element. That's all. Taking 2 mg of copper a day is good health insurance.

Keep in mind that while some people are copper deficient, people with hypertension often have excessive levels of copper. It would take about 15 mg of copper a day for it to become toxic, however, and that is very unlikely.

Dosage

Take 2 mg of copper a day. Copper citrates, oxides, and gluconates are all very absorbable.

GALLIUM

Gallium is a very overlooked element that was one of a few supplements unfortunately banned by the FDA in 2016. The few studies we have on gallium are very positive, however, especially as related to bone metabolism. It is no longer allowed in mineral supplements, even in mere 100 mcg amounts. There should be more research on this important element. Gallium is a vital ultra-trace mineral, and gallium nitrate is a good form to use.

Dosage

Take 100 mcg of gallium a day.

GERMANIUM

Germanium is a very important ultra-trace element, but you will not find it in mineral supplements since the 2016 FDA ban. Clinical human blood studies have proven that germanium is vital to our health, but our food, and the soil our food is grown in, is germanium deficient. Germanium sesquioxide and chelates are safe, but germanium dioxide is not.

Dosage

You only need about 100 mcg a day of ultra-trace elements like germanium. Do not take more than 100 mcg of germanium a day.

IODINE

Iodine is one of two nonmetallic elements you need to supplement (the other nonmetallic element you need is silicon). It is very important to your health. Iodine plays a crucial role in balancing your thyroid metabolism. There are only about 30 mg of iodine in your body, and three-fourths of this is in your thyroid gland. There is just no reason to use iodized salt; we use too much salt in our diets already. This is simply not a good way to get iodine. Surprisingly, regularly eating sea vegetables like kelp, nori, and hijiki (as many Asians do), is not a good idea either. All seaweeds contain extreme amounts of iodine, and overdoses of any mineral unbalance your metabolism. It's important to note that *iodine supplements will not correct thyroid problems* such as hypothyroidism.

Dosage

The RDI of iodine is 150 mcg.

IRON

Iron is the "heme" in hemoglobin, and it's the basic mineral in our blood. Iron deficiency is as common as ever, despite our excessive consumption of red meat. This irony can only be explained by an inability to absorb the iron we need. Excessive iron levels are very rare, and this is due to a metabolic excretion problem, rather than excessive intake. Iron deficiency is as prevalent as ever.

Dosage

Find a good supplement that contains the female RDI of 18 mg or the male RDI of 10 mg. Common sulfates, fumarates, and gluconates are good forms to take.

MAGNESIUM

Magnesium is generally deficient in Western diets because we consume too many refined foods. Whole grains contain plenty of magnesium, but Americans eat a mere one percent whole grains—we should be eating at least 30 percent or more! Many illnesses have been correlated to low levels of magnesium in the blood. If you eat whole grains daily, you simply don't need magnesium supplements.

Dosage

The RDI of magnesium is 400 mg.

MANGANESE

Manganese is a very important mineral for our health, and yet the RDI was only recently established at 2 mg. Whole grains, along with beans and legumes, nuts, and some vegetables, are the major source of manganese. Our refined foods take much of the manganese out of our diets.

There is an abundance of research about the benefits of manganese for our health. For example, our bodies need it for fat metabolism, growth factors, reproduction, muscle coordination, and brain function. Manganese deficiency can result in bone disease, carpal tunnel syndrome, infertility, menopausal problems, arthritis, and osteoporosis.

Dosage

A 2 mg daily supplement of manganese is good health insurance, since we only have around 20 mg of manganese in our bodies. Whole grains, beans, and leafy green vegetables are the best sources of manganese. Sulfates and oxides are good forms to take.

MOLYBDENUM

Molybdenum is safe and nontoxic, even though it is a heavy metal. The research on molybdenum has been more concerned with soils and plants, rather than with animals and humans. Farmers and gardeners, for instance, commonly use molybdenum in their fertilizer and animal feed. Unfortunately, there has been very little research on the relationship between molybdenum deficiency and various diseases and conditions. However, molybdenum is recognized as an important element for bone and joint health, as well as blood sugar metabolism. Anticancer and antitumor properties have been attributed to molybdenum as well.

Dosage

Molybdenum has an RDI of 75 mcg. Common salts are good sources of molybdenum, and you should find this in most all supplement formulas.

NICKEL

Nickel is an ultra-trace element that is often ignored, and 100 mcg a day is all you need. Blood analysis of animals and humans has shown us that nickel is an essential element for our health. There has been little research on the specific benefits of nickel, or the problems caused by nickel deficiency. The research on nickel has been mostly concerned with mineral deficiencies in our soil, and how they affect the growth of our crops.

Not much research has been done on how nickel deficiencies affect the health of livestock and humans. The few studies we have in this area have shown us some very promising things.

For instance, children with very high IQs have higher levels of serum nickel than children with average IQs. Nickel also plays an important role in fertility. Women with low levels of nickel are more likely to experience infertility or hypertension during pregnancy. People are unaware that nickel a very important mineral. You'll rarely ever see this in a mineral supplement.

Dosage

Supplement your diet with 100 mcg of nickel a day. You probably won't see nickel in mineral supplements on the market. Regular salts, such as chlorides and sulfates, are good sources of nickel.

SELENIUM

Selenium had been ignored by nutritionists for decades, but finally the Food and Drug Administration (FDA) has given this essential mineral an official RDI of 70 mcg. Studies show that people with low levels of selenium in their blood are more likely to suffer from cancer, coronary heart disease, and diabetes. Our soils, as well as the heavily refined foods we eat, are very deficient in selenium. Whole grains are the very best source of selenium.

Dosage

Be sure to take your selenium supplement with 200 IU of vitamin E, because selenium and vitamin E work synergistically. Do not exceed a daily intake of more than 200 mcg, as it is a heavy metal and will accumulate in your body. Use a chelate.

SILICON

Sometimes referred to as the "orphan mineral," silicon is another ignored element that is almost never found in mineral supplements. Silicon is the only other nonmetallic element we need besides iodine. The lack of silicon supplements just provides more proof that megacorporations have no research departments, only advertising budgets.

Silica levels in our foods vary so greatly, it is all but impossible to determine which foods are good sources. That said, onions, beets, kale, brown rice, and oats are all fine sources of silicon. Unfortunately, there aren't enough studies on the importance of silicon in our diets. We do know, however, that silicon is a basic building block for our bones, cartilage, and tendons. The science here is most impressive.

We also know that temporarily taking extra silica gel (or silicic acid) has the unique property of absorbing excess aluminum that's in our bodies and helping us excrete it. This is crucial, since excess aluminum is toxic and builds up in the brains of Alzheimer's patients. Americans tend to have high levels of aluminum in their blood. Silicon has many important health benefits, but there need be many more scientific studies on this vital mineral.

Dosage

There is no RDI set for silicon, but 10 mg a day is a safe and effective dose. Plain silica gel is a good, inexpensive source of silicon.

STRONTIUM

Strontium is another very important trace element with very good science behind it. You will rarely find strontium in mineral supplements, but 1,000 mcg (one mg) a day is a good dose. Like silicon, bone and joint health depend on strontium as a building block, and it's also necessary for calcium absorption. No RDI has been set, but science finally recognizes strontium as an essential part of our nutrition.

Dosage

Look for a supplement that has 1,000 mcg (one mg)-strontium chelates and asparates are good choices. Do not confuse this with the radioactive form: strontium-90.

TIN

Another important ultra-trace element, and one that is often ignored, is tin. Common food and soil studies have proven that tin is an essential element, but most of the research on tin has been concerned with its toxicity (from industrial pollution), instead of with its health benefits. Unfortunately, the FDA irrationally limits the RDI of tin to 30 mcg, and it's very difficult to find tin in mineral supplements. Human studies have shown that low blood levels are associated with various illnesses, but more research needs to be done on this subject.

Dosage

Taking 100 mcg of tin a day is a healthy dose, but the FDA limits this to 30 mcg. Regular salts, such as chlorides and sulfates, are good sources of tin, and are easily absorbed by our bodies.

VANADIUM

Vanadium also was also ignored by nutritionists until very recently. There is still no RDI for vanadium, because it is not considered an essential element. Vanadium has been proven a critical mineral for our health in general, and whole grains and seafood are excellent sources of vanadium. Unfortunately, due to our high intake of refined foods, vanadium deficiency is all too common.

There is now very good science on the importance of vanadium. For example, vanadium is extremely important in blood sugar metabolism and diabetes prevention. It also plays a key role in bone, tooth, and cartilage repair and maintenance. Furthermore, vanadium even has anticancer and antitumor properties.

Dosage

Taking one mg of vanadium a day is good, but almost no supplements contain this vital mineral. Do not take more than one to 2 mg a day, as vanadium is toxic at 10 mg. Chelates and sulfates are the best vanadium supplements.

ZINC

Zinc levels are generally low in men with prostate disease. Most people do not get the 15 mg RDI they need from the foods they eat. Zinc is found in whole grains, beans, nuts, and meats, but whole grains and beans are the best sources.

Zinc deficiency is particularly a problem for the poor, the young, the elderly, and alcoholics. There are about 2.5 g of zinc in the human body, half of which is in the muscles. Zinc is necessary for the synthesis of RNA and DNA, growth and development, reproduction, immunity, and many other bodily processes.

Dosage

The RDI for zinc is 15 mg. The usual citrates, oxides, and sulfates all work well as supplements. Even though zinc has a low toxicity level, you should never take more than 50 mg of zinc a day.

CONCLUSION

In the future, it is very possible that we may need other ultra-trace elements such as barium, europium, rubidium, neodymium, praseodymium, thulium, lithium, tungsten, samarium, lanthanum, and yttrium. It is very difficult to determine the effects of these elements, since they are needed in such tiny microgram amounts. *What is all too clear is that the mineral supplements on the market are woefully inadequate.* It will be difficult to find the right supplement mineral supplement, but with this information you can find one. Always read the label! Supplementing your diet with these vital minerals will help set you live a healthy, disease-free life.

5. Beta-Sitosterol and Prostate Health

The most proven effective nutritional supplement for prostate health is a common plant alcohol called beta-sitosterol. Beta-sitosterol is found in literally all of the vegetables you eat, and it is the most prominent plant sterol in nature.

Beta-sitosterol is actually a combination of several sterols, including campesterol, stigmasterol, and brassicasterol. So, we really mean "mixed sterols" when we refer to the term *beta-sitosterol*. It is estimated that Americans consume about 300 mg or less of these mixed plant sterols a day. Vegetarians consume about twice that much.

THE TRUTH ABOUT PLANT STEROL SUPPLEMENTS

Traditionally, herbs such as saw palmetto, Pygeum africanum, nettles, and star grass have been used to treat prostate problems. The trouble with using these herbs is that they contain only a tiny amount (one part per three thousand) of the sterol complex. A typical analysis of saw palmetto, for example, shows that it contains a variety of fatty acids (capric, eicosenoic, lauric, myristic, palmitic, and others), but only minute—and therefore biologically insignificant—traces of sterols and other plant chemicals. These herbal formulas just do not contain any effective amounts of the active ingredients.

You would have to eat a pound of saw palmetto berries in order to obtain a basic dose of 300 mg of phytosterols. Even if you take "10x" extracts of these herbs (with ten times the normal amount sterols), you would still have to eat about two hundred 500 mg capsules, in order to get 300 mg of sterols! Analyses published in *Biochemistry, Gazzetta Chimica Italia, Journal of High Resolution Chromatography, Journal of Pharmacy Science,* and the *Indian Journal of Chemistry* have shown that sterols make up less than one percent of these herbs.

It is obvious that saw palmetto and other such herbs are ineffective, despite their continual promotion by the so-called natural health industry. Even when the product label reads "85 percent fatty acids and sterols," it usually means "nearly all fatty acids and almost no sterols." Choosing the best beta-sitosterol supplement can be tricky, especially with so many ineffective products on the market, so always read the product label carefully before you try a new supplement.

But what about the herbal extracts sold by prescription in Europe? These extracts are standardized by law according to phytosterol content (regardless of its source), and the content is prominently and clearly stated on the label. Whether you buy Permixon in France; Harzol, Tadenan, or Azuprostat in Germany; or Prostaserene in Belgium, these products are all sold according to how much actual sitosterol content they have. Though very expensive, these products are fairly weak. A bottle of sixty tablets of Permixon, for example, containing 30 mg of sterols per tablet, will cost about 50 USD. You would have to take ten tablets a day to get any benefit, which would cost you about 250 USD a month. You can buy a sixty day supply of 300 mg mixed sterols in America for under $10.

It is obvious that such herbs are very uneconomical sources of beta-sitosterol. However, soybeans, sugarcane pulp, and pine oil (tall oil) are all excellent, natural, and inexpensive sources of plant sterols. Many cane-sugar processors now extract the valuable chemicals from the pulp after the sugar is pressed out. Still, only a few companies sell actual beta-sitosterol supplements containing 300 mg or more. Unfortunately, most prostate sup plements contain insufficient amounts. Find a reliable supplement with at least 300 mg of mixed sterols per capsule or tablet.

PROSTATE HEALTH BENEFITS OF PLANT STEROLS

There have been dozens of classic double-blind studies on men regarding the effects of phytosterols on BPH or enlarged prostates. We'll discuss a few of these to give you some examples of the first-rate research that has been done around the world at leading hospitals and clinics.

At Ruhr University Bochum in Herne, Germany (*The Lancet* v 345, 1995), Dr. Berges and his associates studied the effects of pure beta-sitosterol on 200 men over the course of a year. Half of the men received sterols while the other half received a placebo. Dr. Berges and his colleagues concluded, "Significant improvement in symptoms and urinary flow parameters show the effectiveness of beta-sitosterol in the treatment of BPH." While this is one of the most important and well-done experiments on prostate health ever published, there are many other noteworthy studies on this subject.

At the Institute of Clinical Medicine at the University of Rome (*European Urology* v 21, 1992), Dr. Di Silverio and his colleagues studied thirty-five men with BPH for three months, giving half of them beta-sitosterol and half of them a placebo. They concluded, "On the basis of these considerations, monotherapy with a saw palmetto extract may be more favorably accepted, on account of similar clinical results, when compared to the combination therapy cyproterone acetate plus tamoxifen."

A few years later, Doctors Wilt and MacDonald at the University of Rome (*British Journal of Urology* v 83, 1999) gave Permixon to BPH patients with an average age of sixty-eight. Over a ninety-day period, the addition of Permixon to their diets caused a 50 percent drop in their serum dihydrotestosterone (DHT) levels, and a 72 percent boost in their testosterone levels.

So, the sterol therapy actually lowered their DHT levels, as well as helped stop their binding to the prostate. This study provides further proof that testosterone is necessary for healthy prostate metabolism, contrary to what many medical doctors believe.

For some reason, most doctors irrationally feel testosterone is "bad" for prostate health. Hundreds of published clinical studies prove that high testosterone levels are correlated with healthy prostates, while low levels of testosterone cause prostate disease. Doctors usually give prostate cancer patients testosterone deprivation treatments. Instead, they should be raising their patients' testosterone levels. Ninety-five percent of men over the age of fifty already suffer from low testosterone. The serum level of DHT is less important than the level of testosterone itself.

The important issue is how much DHT binds to the prostate. When men don't have enough testosterone to bind to the testosterone receptors on their prostate glands, DHT can bind to them instead. Raising your testosterone levels will prevent DHT from binding to the prostate. Your prostate prefers real testosterone. Phytosterols can help prevent DHT from binding to testosterone receptors. In the same journal, doctors at the Veterans Administration in Minneapolis delivered an extensive review of the research on beta-sitosterol. Going back over thirty years, and including thirty-two references, they concluded that beta-sitosterol has "the greatest efficacy amongst phytotherapeutical substances." Furthermore, they found, "Beta-sitosterol improves urological symptoms and flow measures." Reviews like this condense many studies into one comprehensive presentation, and are most valuable.

At the Hospital Ambroise in Paris (*British Journal of Clinical Pharmacology* v 18, 1984), Dr. Champault and two of his colleagues carried out a classic double-blind study on 110 men, half of whom received a placebo. They concluded, "Thus, as predicted by pharmacological and biochemical studies, four tablets of Permixon daily would appear to be a useful therapeutic tool in the treatment of BPH." Of course, Dr. Champault should have used more beta-sitosterol than that to see even better results.

At the Klinische Endokrinologie in Freiburg, Germany (*Klinische Endokrinologie* v 98, 1980), Dr. Zahradnik and his colleagues demonstrated that Harzol (beta-sitosterol) lowered prostaglandin levels. It has been shown that high prostaglandin levels support tumor growth, so it's important to maintain low levels of prostaglandin.

Doctors at the University of Padova in Italy (*Minerva Urologica e Nefrologica* v 37, 1985) studied the effect of a special high-potency beta-sitosterol extract on men with BPH. Dr. Tasca and his associates measured urine flow, as well as other parameters, in men ranging from ages forty-nine to eighty-one. They compared the sterol results to the effects from the placebo. The men who received beta-sitosterol achieved a much improved urine flow.

In a similar study, Doctor Bassi and his associates at the University of Padova (*Minerva Urologica e Nefrologica* v 39, 1987) analyzed forty BPH patients and the effect of a special high-potency sterol extract. Half the men received the sterol supplement, while half of them received a placebo. The doctors concluded, "The preliminary results demonstrate a significant improvement of the frequency, urgency, dysuria [difficult, painful urination], and urinary flow in patients treated with the active drug."

At the University of Dresden in Germany (*British Journal of Urology* v 80, 1997), the doctors studied 177 men with BPH for six months. Half of the men received a placebo, and half received the prescription extract Azuprostat (beta-sitosterol). To substantiate their research, the doctors cited thirty-two references and carefully screened all the men, who were tested extensively during the study. Dr. Klippel and his colleagues concluded, "These results show that beta-sitosterol is an effective option in the treatment of BPH."

A nine-week double-blind study of fifty men was conducted at the University of Basel in Switzerland (*Urologe A* v 24, 1985). Dr. Vontobel and his colleagues studied a high potency phytosterol extract. They stated, "The use of beta-sitosterol in the evaluation of the objective parameters showed significant differences; the men who received the supplement improved significantly."

At eight different urological clinics in Europe (*Wiener Klinische Wochenschrift* v 102, 1990), a collective study on 263 BPH patients was carried out over a two-month period. The patients were given either Tadenan (beta-sitosterol) or a placebo. This very extensive study concluded, "Treatment with the extract led to a marked clinical improvement. A comparison of the quantitative parameters showed a significant difference between the treated group and the placebo group, with respect to therapeutic response." Doctors involved in this study concluded that phytosterols are the most promising medical therapy for treating prostate disease.

A study on twenty-three patients was done at the Urological Clinic of Krankenhaus in Germany (*Medizinische Klinik* v 77, 1982). Over a two-month period, Dr. Szutrely gave patients with BPH either Harzol (beta-sitosterol) or a placebo. He measured their prostates with ultrasound equipment before and after treatment. He found, "Within the scope of a controlled double blind study to demonstrate the effect of conservative therapy of benign prostatic hyperplasia (BPH) with Harzol, ultrasonic examination of the prostate adenoma (a benign tumor) was carried out on twenty-three patients before and after therapy, with the trial preparation of a placebo. Within a two-month treatment with Harzol there was a significant change in echo structure of the prostate adenoma. This is interpreted as a reduction in the interstitial formation of edema (excess accumulation of fluid)."

A unique review by Dr. Wilt at the Department of Veterans Affairs (*Journal of the American Medical Association* v 280, 1998) of prostate studies examined eighteen different international trials, involving 2,939 men with BPH, that were conducted over a thirty-one-year period. The participants in these trials were given strong extracts of saw palmetto that had been standardized for sterol content. After reviewing all these studies, Dr. Wilt and researchers announced, "The evidence suggests that Serenoa repens (saw palmetto) extract improves urologic symptoms and flow measures." Again, this was based on eighteen published studies.

Another interesting review was conducted by the Department of Urology at the University of Glasgow in Scotland (*British Journal of Urology* v 78, 1996). Dr. Buck wrote a twelve-page review of phytosterol based prostate supplements. In the review, Dr. Buck discusses the biological basis of prostate illness. He documents his report by citing fifty-nine published international studies. His conclusions of the efficacy of plant sterols are well founded.

In Belgium, Dr. Braekman performed a study at the University of Brussels (*Current Therapeutic Research* v 55, 1994), using Prostaserene (beta-sitosterol). Over a period of three months, some 505 BPH patients were given a twice-daily dose of Prostaserene. Dr. Braekman's observations led him to conclude, "Traditional parameters for quantifying prostatism, such as the International Prostate Symptom Score, the quality-of-life score, urinary flow rates, residual urinary volume, and prostate size were found to be significantly improved after only forty-five days of treatment. After ninety days of treatment, a majority of patients (88 percent) and treating physicians (88 percent) considered the therapy effective."

There is another fine review on the effects of plant sterols and BPH from the University of Connecticut (*Pharmacotherapy* v 22, 2002). Dr. Coleman and his colleagues agreed, "In men with BPH, evidence suggests that the agents improve urologic symptoms and flow measures to a greater extent than placebo and to a similar extent as finasteride. Beta-sitosterols also are efficacious in the treatment of BPH, improving urinary symptoms and flow measures in placebo-controlled clinical trials. Phytosterols improved lower urinary tract symptoms (LUTS) and urinary flow measures in numerous clinical trials." The researchers were also very concerned with measuring patients' quality of life (QOL) and concluded, "Based on the studies reviewed, phytosterols are generally well tolerated and potentially effective in treating symptoms of BPH and improving quality of life." This was defined by the International Prostate Symptom Score (IPSS), which was developed in 1993 and is considered to be the gold standard for urological symptoms.

In May 2000, Dr. Berges and his associates at Ruhr University Bochum in Bochum, Germany published another study on beta-sitosterol (*British Journal of Urology* v 85, 2000). This time, they carried out a long-term study in order to prove the lasting effects of plant sterol therapy on BPH. In a classic double-blind study, conducted over an eighteen-month period, they measured many basic indexes (such as the IPSS and urine flow) to show in detail how the men fared. While men given only a placebo grew worse with time, those men given sterols improved in all measured ways. Dr. Berges and his colleagues concluded, "The beneficial effects of sterol treatment were maintained for eighteen months." Clearly, plant sterols are an effective treatment for BPH, even over long periods of time.

CONCLUSION

These are only a few of the many plant sterol studies that have appeared in major medical journals over the last thirty years. Each study shows that mixed phytosterols are the active ingredient in popular herbs, such as saw palmetto. Most of the prostate supplements sold in America have few sterols in them. Just read the label to see what is in there. You must get at least 300 mg in each capsule or tablet—not "per dose." There are good supplements out there if you just look. Mixed plant sterols are the most effective prostate support known. Worldwide studies, at reputable hospitals and clinics, have all confirmed that phytosterols reduce prostate enlargement in men suffering from BPH. No matter how old you are, no matter how sick, beta-sitosterol can improve your health.

6. Other Benefits of Phytosterols

Beta-sitosterol is the most important supplement to take for prostate health, but it has many other benefits as a daily supplement. Women, for example, should take sterols to protect against breast cancer and other breast conditions. Breast cancer is the female equivalent of prostate cancer, with the very same causes and the very same cures.

Plant sterols can also be used to help treat a wide range of conditions, including high cholesterol, various cancers, diabetes, ulcers, inflammation, poor blood clotting, poor blood parameters, and others. Sterols have antioxidant, antibacterial, antiviral, antimicrobial, and anti-infective properties as well. Everyone over the age of forty should be taking a supplement of at least 300 mg of mixed sterols a day.

PLANT STEROLS CAN LOWER YOUR CHOLESTEROL

Another important benefit of plant sterols is that they can help lower cholesterol and triglyceride levels. Coronary heart disease is the biggest killer worldwide by far. Your cholesterol and triglyceride levels are the two most important diagnostic indicators of your heart and artery health. The scientific studies on cholesterol and plant sterols actually go back fifty years, but the general public (and most medical professionals) remains unaware of this. Please read my book, *Lower Cholesterol Without Drugs.*

At McGill University in Montreal (*Canadian Journal of Physiology* v 75, 1997), a review of decades of scientific literature on beta-sitosterol was conducted. Researchers concluded that the "addition to diet of phytosterols represents an effective means of improving circulating lipid profiles to reduce risk of coronary heart disease." In another study from McGill University (*Metabolism, Clinical & Experimental* v 47, 1998), patients were given plant sterols for just ten days. This was a strict placebo-controlled study in which the patients otherwise continued their normal diets. Total and LDL cholesterol levels were lowered significantly in just ten days.

Perhaps the best phytosterol review of all is from the University of British Columbia (the *American Journal of Medicine* v 107, 1999). This study included eighty-six clinical references dating back to 1951. Researchers discovered that "In sixteen recently published human studies that used phytosterols to decrease plasma cholesterol levels in a total of 590 subjects, phytosterol therapy was accompanied by an average 10 percent decrease in total cholesterol and 13 percent decrease in LDL cholesterol." Moreover, the reviewers noticed an interesting trend in the clinical studies: The worse the diet, the greater the patients' health would improve, and the better the results! This is a stunning review!

At Uppsala University in Sweden (*European Heart Journal* Supp. 1, 1999), volunteers were given mixed plant sterols in conjunction with a low-fat, cholesterol-lowering diet. A low-fat diet greatly enhances the beneficial effects of phytosterols. In less than a month, the men and women lowered their total cholesterol a full 15 percent and their LDL cholesterol an amazing 19 percent! This study shows that drugs are not necessary at all. A combination of plant sterols and better food choices—even with no exercise—produced very dramatic results in less than thirty days. This is an infinitely better choice than statins.

PHYTOSTEROLS CAN HELP
TREAT AND PREVENT CANCER

People who eat more vegetables, and therefore more plant sterols, have lower rates of every known cancer. Most of these studies are being done on animals. At Virginia Polytech Institute (*Cancer Research* v 34, 1974), doctors found that plant sterols are an important factor in preventing colon cancer. The sterols help balance and improve the intestinal flora.

Another study on colon cancer was conducted at the Sloan-Kettering Cancer Institute (*Journal of Cancer Research* v 103, 1982). Merely feeding rats sterols reduced tumor growth and prevented new tumors from growing. Additionally, at Wayne State University (the *Journal of the National Cancer Institute* v 66, 1982) sterols were shown to help prevent intestinal cancer in rats.

And at Nihon University in Japan (*Oncology* v 49, 1991) sterols were shown to inhibit skin cancer in mice when researchers simply applied it to the rats' skin. At the State University of New York at Buffalo (*International Journal of Molecular Medicine* v 5, 2000), beta-sitosterol was found to inhibit both prostate and breast cancer cells. Another fine review from the University of Buffalo (*Journal of Nutrition* v 130, 2000) revealed that phytosterols in general can help prevent and treat various cancers. This study was complete with a full forty-three references and was most impressive.

PHYTOSTEROLS CAN HELP
CURE BLOOD SUGAR DISORDERS

Diabetes, hyperglycemia, hyperinsulinemia, and insulin resistance are now epidemics in Western countries. *One in three American children will now grow up diabetic.* High blood sugar levels (i.e., over 100) characterize type 2 diabetes. Phytosterol supplementation should be part of a comprehensive program to prevent and treat all blood sugar and insulin conditions.

At Dhaka University in Bangladesh (*Pure & Applied Chemistry* v 66, 1994), scientists discovered that phytosterols had hypoglycemic properties that helped lower blood sugar levels in diabetic rats. A similar study at Shiga University in Japan (*Biochemical Biophysical Research Communications* v 186, 1992) confirmed that phytosterols can lower blood sugar levels in diabetic rats. Furthermore, Drs. Ivora and D'Ocon (*Archives Internationales de Pharmacodynamie et de Therapie* v 296, 1988) found that sterols fed to hyperglycemic rats lowered their blood sugar levels; they concluded, "These results indicate a possible anti-hyperglycemic use for the phytosterols in the prevention and treatment of diabetic and pre-diabetic conditions." Soon, we'll have human studies to verify what we already know from animal studies. Read my book, *The Natural Diabetes Cure.*

PHYTOSTEROLS CAN TREAT AND PREVENT STOMACH ULCERS

Stomach ulcers are now very common in America. At West China University (*Huaxi Yike Daxue Xeubao* v 23, 1992), plant sterols exhibited anti-ulcer properties in rats. The sterols dramatically improved chronic gastric ulcers. A few years later, in another study at West China University (*Huaxi Yaoxue Zazhi* v 11, 1996), the same anti-ulcer properties were demonstrated in experimental laboratory animals.

Back in the United States, at the University of Texas (*Digestive Science* v 35, 1990), doctors reduced and eliminated gastric ulceration in rats by simply feeding the animals phytosterols. Of their research, the doctors declared, "The results suggest that the sterols may promote the packing of adjacent unsaturated phospholipids . . . to provide the mucosa with protection against luminal acid." Why aren't people being studied as well?

PHYTOSTEROLS CAN REDUCE INFLAMMATION

Many illnesses involve chronic inflammation, which is basically a complex biological response of our vascular tissues to harmful stimuli. Inflammation results in redness, heat, swelling, and pain, but plant sterols have shown good anti-inflammatory properties. At the Universidade Federal de Santa Catarina in Brazil (*Planta Medica* v 61, 1995), mice were given sterols and then tested for inflammation markers. The mice "exhibited significant analgesic action" and reduced pain from inflammation.

Published in the very same journal (*Planta Medica* v 39, 1980), a study conducted at King George's Medical College in India found "potent anti-inflammatory, and analgesic (pain reducing), and anti-pyretic (fever reducing) properties" for sterols. Rats given the sterols in their food achieved dramatic results, and it was concluded, "Sterols possess highly potent anti-inflammatory and antipyretic actions, suggesting its application to human medicine." Finally, in a study at the University of Naples in Italy (*Bulletin of the Italian Society of Biology* v 65, 1989), researchers stated that plant sterols "exhibit moderate anti-inflammatory properties." Doctors and scientists all over the world agree that phytosterols reduce inflammation, a major cause of many illnesses.

PHYTOSTEROLS CAN HELP PREVENT BLOOD CLOTS

What could be more important that the quality of our blood? Plant sterols have been shown to dramatically improve many common blood parameters. At the Tokyo Institute of Technology (*Tanpakushitsu Kahusan Koso* v 30, 1985), doctors published a review—with no less than eighty-nine references—showing the benefits of beta-sitosterol on various blood parameters. In another comprehensive review at the same institute (*Sogo Rinsho* v 34, 1985), plant sterols were again proven to improve blood parameters. Indeed, a third study at the Tokyo Institute (*Medical Philosophy* v 5, 1986) confirmed the results of the first two reviews. With these extensive studies, researchers were looking for a way to prevent blood diseases such as thrombosis (blood clot formation).

At the Erfurt Medical Academy in Germany (*Folia Haematology* v 115, 1988), scientists discovered further benefits for blood health by simply feeding sterols to laboratory animals. And at Aga Khan University in Pakistan (*Biochemical Society Transactions* v 21, 1993,) even more benefits for blood health were exhibited, including anti-inflammatory and antiplatelet properties.

The best study on the benefits of plant sterols on blood parameters was conducted at the University of Stellenbosch in South Africa (the *International Journal of Immunopharmacology* v 18, 1996). There, real human blood cells were analyzed, and various blood cell parameters were very much improved. What's more, the scientists in Stellenbosch provided forty-two full references along with their findings. This research on plant sterols has very important implications for human health, particularly in the prevention and cure of blood clots. Our blood is literally our life stream.

CONCLUSION

There are many other studies we could quote to show the varied benefits of sterols, but even after looking only at those examples listed above, it is obvious that beta-sitosterol is an extremely important part of your diet. Most people do not eat enough vegetables, so they do not get the sterols they need. Be sure to take 300 to 600 mg a day of mixed sterols to improve not only your prostate health, but also your health in general.

7. Curing Prostatitis and Prostate Cancer

Along with BPH, prostatitis and cancer of the prostate are the two most common forms of prostate disease. These three conditions affect millions of men every year, and, unfortunately, most of these men do not receive the proper treatments. Most medical doctors today treat prostate disease with hormone therapy, surgery, drugs, and radiation. The truth is, there are much safer and more effective ways to cure prostate disease. This chapter discusses how to prevent, treat, and ultimately cure prostatitis and prostate cancer.

PROSTATITIS

Prostatitis is the chronic inflammation of the prostate gland. All too common in western countries, but rare in rural regions of Asia, prostatitis can be a hard-to-cure and very painful, debilitating condition. This inflammation is due to low immunity in the reproductive area. Many factors contribute to low immunity, but poor diet and lifestyle is the main cause. *Ninety percent of our immunity comes from our digestive system.*

Americans eat twice as many calories as they need—a full 40 percent fat calories, twice the necessary protein, 160 pounds of various sugars, and only one percent whole grains. Other factors contributing to low immunity include hormone imbalance, stress (physical and emotional), lack of exercise, mineral deficiency, taking prescription or recreational drugs, alcohol use, smoking, and caffeine. When your immunity is impaired, your body cannot effectively fight off illnesses and cure itself. Attacks of prostatitis can be triggered by various factors including anal intercourse (heterosexual or homosexual), urethritis (urinary tract infections), cystitis (bladder infections) or postsurgical complications.

Preventing Prostatitis

How can you strengthen your immunity? With a total program of diet and lifestyle. Nothing less. Strengthen your digestive system. The main thing is to eat well. Diet is everything.

Read my book *Macrobiotics for Everyone.* Take proven supplements. Balance your basic hormones. Exercise. Fast one day every week. Do not take prescription or recreational drugs, except for short-term emergencies. Stop drinking alcohol and caffeine. Strengthen your digestive system, and you'll enhance your immune system. Stop smoking and using tobacco. Eat two meals a day. Eat only macrobiotic food. Don't eat out, and pack your lunch for work. Take acidophilus and FOS in the morning, and then again in the evening. Buy bulk glutamine and take one tablespoon a day. Take two aloe vera capsules a day for six months.

Follow this regimen and your digestive system will be renewed. You can also rejuvenate your liver by taking 3 g (six capsules) of trimethylglycine (TMG) a day for six months. Your liver is essential to your digestion. Strengthening your immunity is going to take time and patience, but you will get results every month. You are going to have to treat yourself with a total program of diet and lifestyle if you want to cure an inflamed prostate gland and keep it cured. Prostatitis is actually more difficult to cure than outright prostate cancer, since it is chronic and due to lowered immunity. Patience and determination will help you achieve this.

Detecting and Treating Prostatitis

Most cases of prostatitis are simply the chronic variety with moderate swelling, inflammation, and discomfort. Acute chronic prostatitis is a much more dangerous affair. Men can suffer from chills, fever, pain in the reproductive area, burning urination, and frequent urination. This can easily be diagnosed by finding white blood cells and bacteria in the urine.

There are many types of bacteria that cause prostatitis, such as E. coli, klebsiella, and proteus. The usual medical treatment is powerful bactericidal antibiotics, such as doxycycline, that kill the bacteria outright. (Bacteriostatic antibiotics like tetracycline merely slow down bacterial growth.) The bacteria are not causing the problem at all. They are a symptom, not a cause, per se. The bacteria can only grow because of an impaired immune system that would normally stop their development.

Such treatments, of course, are purely symptomatic, and do nothing to deal with the cause of the bacterial assault. In fact, these antibiotics harm the digestive system and kill off the good digestive bacteria in our stomach and intestines. The patient ends up in worse shape than ever. Yet such antibiotic therapy often is routinely used. Often patients who receive no medical treatment at all recover just as quickly as those who do. Doctors have also resorted to prescribing alpha-blockers, anti-inflammatories, physiotherapy, and even surgery, all to no avail.

There is also a condition called *nonbacterial prostatitis,* in which no invading bacteria can be determined in the urine. The symptoms here are blood in semen, blood in urine, pain in the genital area, frequent urination, burning urination, weak urine stream, pain with ejaculation, and pain during bowel movements. Taking antibiotics in such cases is useless. Doctors can do nothing here but take your money and worsen your health with worthless toxic prescription drugs.

Facing the Facts

Prostatitis, or any slight infection of the prostate, can falsely raise your prostate-specific antigen (PSA) levels. This often leads to damaging and very unnecessary biopsies. This is just further proof that the PSA is not an accurate diagnostic tool at all and should be abandoned. More and more researchers are admitting the PSA is inaccurate, misleading, and should be dropped. The inventor of this test said it is a waste of time and money. Biopsies are never called for, and only about one quarter of men who get them have cancer. Biopsies only stimulate malignancy.

Unfortunately, there is very, very little scientific research on the natural treatment of prostatitis. The only research available is primarily concerned with using dangerous prescription drugs to cover up the symptoms of disease. What little research there is on natural cures, however, is all very promising. At the Institute for Male Urology in California (*Urology* v 54, 1999) a double-blind study was done. Men with prostatitis were given 500 mg of quercetin twice a day for a month, though half of them were really given a placebo. The men who received the quercetin improved their health by 25 percent, without any change to diet or lifestyle. The men who received the placebo did not experience any improvement in their disease.

A similar study using quercetin was conducted at the University of California at Los Angeles Harbor Medical Center (*Journal of the American Nutraceutical Association* v 2, 1999), and this clinical trial also produced positive results. Just taking a natural antioxidant like quercetin helps cure prostatitis. Imagine the results you could have if you took quercetin and other supplements in conjunction with a total program of diet and lifestyle.

PROSTATE CANCER

Prostate cancer is the leading cancer for American men, and the second leading cause of cancer mortality. Most men will eventually have cancer cells in their prostate, unless they change their diet and lifestyle. Prostate cancer is clearly caused by poor diet and lifestyle. This is the mirror image of breast cancer in

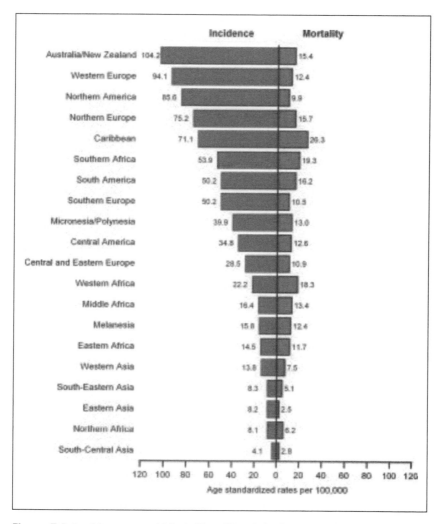

Figure 7.1. Incidence and Mortality of Prostate Cancer in Developed and Undeveloped Regions. This figure compares the incidence of prostate cancer across twenty different regions, including both developed and undeveloped parts of the world. Note that North America has one of the highest rates of prostate cancer. Those in less industrialized regions of the world (who consume less fatty and highly-processed foods) are much less likely to develop prostate cancer.

women, with the same causes and natural cures. Saturated animal fat is the main cause of prostate (and breast) cancer, plain and simple. Just look at Figure 7.1, Incidence and Mortality of Prostate Cancer in Developed and Undeveloped Regions. There is a twenty-five times difference between the lowest and the highest rates, and this is due to diet and lifestyle. This chart proves diet and lifestyle is the main cause.

Preventing Prostate Cancer

This is a very slow-growing cancer. One in six American men over fifty is walking around with cancer cells in his prostate gland. Early detection is not the answer at all. *Prevention is the answer.* Diet and lifestyle are the answer. Taking meat, poultry, eggs, and dairy foods out of your diet is the first step.

Detecting and Treating the Disease

There are no symptoms in the beginning. *The PSA test is not reliable at all.* Don't even waste your time—the inventor of this test even said it should be dropped. Get a sonogram, an MRI, or even a color Doppler ultrasound to actually see an electronic photograph of your prostate gland. Never get an x-ray of any kind. *Never, ever get a biopsy for any reason.* Biopsies only stimulate cancer growth and should not be done. The symptoms do not show up until the cancer is very advanced. Burning urination, difficult urination, and blood in the urine can be signs of cancer, or signs of mere BPH. In its last stages, cancer can produce symptoms such as fatigue, malaise, weight loss, abdominal pain, back and chest pain, and jaundice.

The prostate cancer industry is about money, money, and more money. The standard treatments are incredibly expensive, yet they merely cover up the symptoms, and leave the cause intact. Surgery, radiation, drugs, and chemotherapy leave the patient with no quality of life at all. Diapers and impotence are the usual outcome, and then the poor man will typically die anyway. The medical treatments also leave you bankrupt.

Yes, prostate cancer can be cured naturally, without resorting to surgery, radiation, drugs or chemotherapy. Prostate cancer may actually be cured by diet alone. As you recall from Chapter 1, the author and actor Dirk Benedict (*The A-Team*) got prostate cancer in his thirties, at the height of his career. He went on a macrobiotic diet and stopped eating meat, poultry, eggs, dairy, refined foods, tropical foods, alcohol, coffee, and sugars of any kind. Of course, Dirk did not have the many supplements and hormones we have now.

The doctors wanted to castrate him, which meant he would die anyway, and with a terrible quality of life. Dirk thought about this option, and decided that the whole grain diet, and living another fifty years, sounded better than dying a painful and premature death, with no testicles. He turned his back on the doctors completely and refused all medical treatments. Within seven months Dirk knew he was basically well, and would soon be completely cancer-free. Over thirty years later, Dirk is happy and healthy. His memoir, *Confessions of a Kamikaze Cowboy*, is an inspiring book and important to read. Other great books on this subject include Anthony Sattarilo's *Recalled By Life* (out of print, but at libraries), Mina Dobic's *My Beautiful Life*, and Elaine Nussbaum's *Recovery From Cancer*.

The most important factor in curing prostate cancer, or any other cancer, is to change your diet and lifestyle. Stop eating eggs, dairy, poultry, meat, and sugars of any kind (even honey, stevia, and maple syrup). Avoid tropical foods, coffee, hydrogenated oils, preservatives and chemicals, and refined foods. Don't smoke, use caffeine, take prescription or recreational drugs, or drink alcohol. A diet based on whole grains, beans, most vegetables, some local fruit, good soups and salads, and small amounts of seafood (if you don't want to be a vegetarian) is the way to cure yourself. There are various books available on the macrobiotic diet, and there are some good authors out there who have written books on macrobiotics. Unfortunately, the vast majority of natural diet books are not good at all—to put it mildly.

As discussed earlier, whole grains such as rice, wheat, buck-wheat, millet, barley, corn, and oats are literally the staff of life. They have been the dietary basis of most cultures for thousands of years. Eating well also means eating low-fat, low-calorie foods, and, as stated in Chapter 1, researchers at the Hutchinson Cancer Center (*Cancer Epidemiology Biomarkers Preview* v 11, 2002) have shown that low-calorie diets help cure prostate cancer in men.

After you have changed your diet, another important thing to do is to take the proven supplements for your general health. Nothing can compensate for not eating well. The supplements recommended in this book are safe, natural, inexpensive, effective, and scientifically proven to support good prostate health.

Fasting is another powerful treatment for healing cancer. Fasting just one day per week (supper one day to supper the next day, drinking only water) can change your health completely. It is literally *the* most powerful healing method known. Some fine books on fasting have been written by Paul Bragg, Joel Fuhrman, Eve Adamson, Nathaniel Bronner, and Allan Cott.

Please remember that true fasting means nothing but water. If you feel you can't fast and go without food, then go on a diet of, say, only brown rice for a period of time. You can also go on a low-calorie, soup-only diet. Soon you will be able to fast one day a week with no problem. People think of fasting as starvation, deprivation, and hunger. Actually, hunger pangs generally go away after the second day, and a feeling of lightness, elation, and joy takes over. Besides being a powerful healing method, fasting also develops character and spirituality.

The another step in curing your prostate cancer is hormone balancing. The prostate is strongly hormone-controlled. Saliva and blood spot testing of hormones is the greatest medical break-through in the last decade. Most of the public is still completely unaware of it, as are medical professionals. Doctors rarely test hormone levels, and have little knowledge of how to do this properly. This includes endocrinologists and holistic doctors.

Hormones are very powerful, are not to be used casually, and should not be taken without first testing your levels. Hormone testing will become very mainstream in the near future. DHEA, testosterone, pregnenolone, progesterone, estradiol, estrone, melatonin, and T3/T4 thyroid levels are all critical to good prostate health. If you wish to maintain the youthful hormone levels you had in your thirties, you can use a hormone supplement and monitor your levels annually, but we will discuss hormone balancing in greater detail in the next chapters.

Affirmative prayer is also effective if you have any religious or spiritual orientation. It is the sincerity of your prayer that counts. Faith is simply trust in the unknown, and trust can and does move mountains. Affirmative prayer works.

A theory called "complementary medicine," uses both conventional allopathic (which tends to treat only the symptoms) and natural (which treats only the cause) medicines, has been popularized. However, you cannot go north and south at the same time, and you cannot successfully use opposing methods of healing. The best way to get well is to use allopathic medicine only for the effective diagnostic techniques it employs. You then have a choice of completely avoiding radiation, chemotherapy, prescription drugs, and surgery. These medical methods merely disguise your symptoms and ignore the causes of your illness.

Use natural treatments to deal with the very cause of your illness. Treat your entire body. Surgery, radiation, drugs, and chemotherapy cannot be reversed. The damage is permanent and cannot be undone.

Facing the Facts

Simply changing your diet and lifestyle may not seem like a very effective treatment plan for prostate cancer, but the fact is, it works. Below are just two accounts—out of dozens—from men who have completely cured themselves of prostate cancer with diet and supplements, and *without* surgery, radiation, or prescriptions drugs.

A classic success story of naturally healing prostate cancer comes from my friend Laddie in 1996. In his fifties, he was diagnosed with prostate cancer and told he would be dead in five years. He would rather die than undergo such torture. His wife was determined not to be a widow, and looked into the natural healing of cancer. She read up on macrobiotics, and immediately put him on a diet of whole grains, beans, most vegetables, local fruits, and some seafood. All his life, Laddie had eaten meat, eggs, poultry, dairy, sugar, alcohol, coffee, and refined foods— the usual American diet. He completely changed his diet and lifestyle.

Taking supplements was the easy part. They were a fraction of the cost of the toxic prescription drugs. He took melatonin and pregnenolone, and used transdermal progesterone cream daily. His thyroid was fine. Saliva testing showed his testosterone and DHEA levels were both low. Laddie went against the advice of his doctor, and took both testosterone and DHEA.

Laddie had never gone without food for more than twelve hours in his life, but he started fasting for twenty-four hours weekly. He even did the monthly two day fasts. He knew he was getting well because he *felt* better. Healthy people feel good. You could just look at him and see he was getting healthier month-by-month. His friends and relatives felt pity for him, and thought he was in extreme denial.

Laddie lost weight, his complexion became clearer, he had more energy, and simply looked and felt better. His original doctor became very upset as he grew healthier and healthier every month, refusing all traditional medical treatments. He told the doctor he had raised his testosterone levels, and was taking four other natural hormones. The doctor became so frustrated that he stopped seeing him, and referred him to a colleague!

After less than eight months, Laddie knew in his heart he was well. He had never felt or looked better in his life. He got a sonogram, which verified he was cured. His second doctor confirmed this. Today, he is in his seventies and is a happy, healthy, and thankful man. He eats well, takes his supplements and hormones, and fasts once a week to celebrate being alive. He expects to live into his nineties.

Bob Young was a seventy-year-old, blind, black jazz musician who lived in New Jersey. His is another success story about using natural methods to heal prostate cancer. After his diagnosis, Bob refused the conventional medical treatments. He heard one of my radio shows and called me at home. Since he couldn't read, his aides read him my books regularly. He changed his diet and quit eating meat, eggs, poultry, and all dairy products. He started eating whole grains and other natural foods. He took all the suggested supplements and tested his basic hormones.

Unlike Laddie's medical doctor, Bob's doctor was very supportive of his natural treatment, and helped him test his hormones. It took two years because of his advanced, long-term tumor growth and his age. Bob finally was diagnosed cancer-free, both by MRI and sonogram. He continued his natural food diet, took his supplements and hormones, and fasted. He played in his jazz band weekly. If an elderly blind man can cure his cancer by changing his lifestyle, then you can, too. Bob was an inspiration to anyone with a serious illness. He died of natural causes at eighty-four.

There are other true-life stories of men who cured prostate cancer naturally on our website library, which you can find at www.youngagain.org. Remember, you can cure your prostate cancer in only one year just by changing your diet and lifestyle. All Seven Steps are outlined at the end of this book (page 119).

CONCLUSION

The scientists of the world should do a lot more research on natural cures—not only for prostatitis and prostate cancer, but also for BPH. Unfortunately, there is just no profit in studying inexpensive, unpatented, nonprescription supplements and hormones, much less diet and lifestyle. The profits come from studying expensive prescription drugs, so that is where most all of the research is going.

Nevertheless, now that you know how to effectively cure your prostatitis, or your prostate cancer, you can look forward to a longer, happier life. You don't have to be one of those men who suffers through hormone therapy, surgery, or chemo-therapy. You can improve your health significantly by simply changing your diet and lifestyle. Make better food choices, take the supplements, balance your hormones, fast weekly, stop any bad habits, exercise, and do not take prescription drugs.

8. Your Basic Hormones

The prostate gland is very much influenced by your hormones. It is vital that you have youthful levels of your basic hormones. In this chapter, we will discuss progesterone, DHEA, melatonin, pregnenolone, progesterone, human growth hormone, T3 and T4, insulin, and cortisol. There is a complete list of basic hormones below. Note that estrogens and testosterone are more fully covered in later chapters.

The Basic Hormones in Your Body

This chapter focuses on several hormones that are important to the well-being of your prostate. Below, you'll find a list of *all* the basic hormones necessary for prostate health.

- ☐ Cortisol
- ☐ Dehydroepiandrosterone (DHEA)
- ☐ Estradiol
- ☐ Estrone
- ☐ Human Growth Hormone (HGH)
- ☐ Insulin
- ☐ Melatonin
- ☐ Pregnenolone
- ☐ Progesterone
- ☐ Testosterone
- ☐ Thyroxine (T4)
- ☐ Triiodothyronine (T3)

PROGESTERONE

Progesterone is thought of as a female hormone, but it actually protects both men and women from excess estrogen. Men need progesterone in their bodies, too, only in smaller amounts than women. The estrogens estradiol and estrone are the feminizing hormones in men, and it is progesterone that is the natural antagonist to them. Excessive estrogen levels in men over fifty cause cancer, breast growth, obesity, and other health problems, but progesterone can help inhibit estrogens.

Nature has given progesterone to both men and women in order to balance and offset the strong effects of estrogen. Men, of course, have naturally lower levels of progesterone than women, so they need less supplementation. Be careful not to confuse real, natural progesterone with progestins (synthetic analogs), like Provera, which have serious side effects. Progestins do not have the advantages of natural progesterone.

Men have specific progesterone receptors on their prostates, so clearly this requires progesterone. Yet, urologists and endocrinologists are blind to such well-established scientific facts. This was demonstrated almost forty years ago at Flinders Medical Center in Australia (*Journal of Steroid Biochemistry* v 12, 1980). The doctors recommended progesterone therapy for prostate disease. In the book *Progesterone and Progestins* (Raven Press 1983), the doctors at Service de Medicale in Paris noted that progesterone was vital for proper prostate health. Progesterone protects men from both estrogen dominance and overactivity of 5-alpha reductase. *Your prostate needs progesterone to be healthy.*

Let's quickly discuss the research that shows progesterone opposes and balances excess estrogen, and is a powerful 5-alpha-reductase inhibitor. Progesterone helps prevent the conversion of beneficial testosterone into dihydrotestosterone (DHT). High levels of DHT are one cause of prostate disease. Your prostate will accept DHT instead of real testosterone if your levels are low. Men over fifty only have about half the testosterone they should. Moreover, they also generally have very high levels of both estradiol and estrone.

The best study on progesterone was conducted over forty years ago at the Faculty of Medicine in Paris (*Journal of Clinical Endocrinology and Metabolism* v 38, 1974). Men were given real transdermal progesterone (groundbreaking at the time), which dramatically inhibited the conversion of testosterone into DHT. The researchers recommended progesterone as a standard therapy for men with prostate disease. This is an important and powerful study, but modern day urologists have simply ignored it. There are many, many animal and cell studies on the benefits of progesterone for prostate disease, but almost no human studies. Since then, there been no more human studies using transdermal progesterone. Instead, doctors are studying very profitable toxic, dangerous, ineffective, and expensive patentable prescription drugs.

The Center for Drug Research in India performed four different studies that all showed how progesterone shrank enlarged rat prostates, and moderated the stimulating effects of estrogen. The main study was published over forty years ago in *Endokrinologie* (v 55, 1970) Just giving progesterone to rats with BPH resulted in significantly reduced prostate volumes—and in only thirty days. This is nothing less than amazing. Only thirty days! Well-done animal studies like this are very important precursors to human studies. There are many such studies in the scientific literature, but where are the human studies?

At Montreal General Hospital (*Journal of Clinical Endocrinology and Metabolism* v 39, 1974), researchers showed that progesterone strongly inhibited DHT formation in men. "The ability of progesterone to inhibit DHT formation represents one mode of action which may account at least in part for their efficacy in treating BHP." This happened over forty years ago.

At the Institute of Clinical Chemistry in Germany (*Prostate* v 6, 1985), doctors discovered that progesterone inhibited 5-alpha reductase in human prostates. This is what converts "good" testosterone into "bad" DHT. Researchers at St. George's Hospital in London found the same effect (*Journal of Endocrinology* v 63, 1974). Progesterone was dramatically effective in inhibiting 5-alpha reductase and the conversion of testosterone into DHT. Similar results were demonstrated at the University of Mainze in Germany (*Journal of Steroid Biochemistry* v 6, 1975).

Dosage

You do not have to test your progesterone levels. Saliva testing does not work, as progesterone is fat-soluble. Progesterone is very poorly absorbed orally. If taken by mouth, it is broken down into unwanted metabolites. Fortunately, progesterone is readily absorbed through the skin into the bloodstream; therefore, transdermal creams are very practical and effective. Find a good brand that contains 1,000 mg of natural, pharmaceutical grade (USP) progesterone per two-ounce jar (500 mg per ounce). This should be stated clearly on the label.

Apply one-eighth of a teaspoon of the cream on your inner wrist (or any thin skin) five days a week. This allows the progesterone to enter the bloodstream, and reach the prostate receptors. Just one-eighth of a teaspoon provides about 7 mg, of which about 2 mg should be absorbed into your system. Progesterone is completely nontoxic and very safe, especially in these small amounts.

DEHYDROEPIANDROSTERONE (DHEA)

DHEA is the second-most important androgen for prostate health after testosterone. DHEA is very important for male sexual and urological health. Men with erectile dysfunction often suffer from low levels of DHEA, and need supplementation. DHEA is called the "life extension hormone" for good reason. Many diseases, including coronary heart disease, show evidence of low levels of DHEA in patients. DHEA levels also fall as we age, as you can see from Figure 8.1, *DHEA Sulfate Levels Throughout Life.*

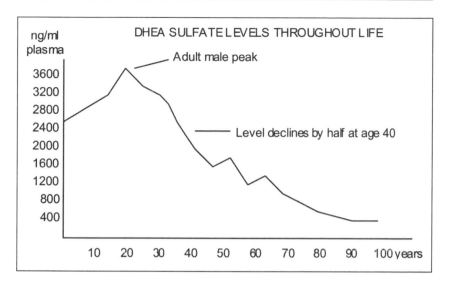

Figure 8.1. DHEA Sulfate Levels Throughout Life. This figure depicts the average man's DHEA sulfate levels throughout his life. Note that levels usually peak around age twenty. And by the time he turns forty, a man's DHEA levels are typically only half what they were at his physical peak.

Men with prostate cancer were found to have decidedly lower DHEA levels than healthy controls (*Urology Times* v 26, 1998). Similarly, at Johns Hopkins University, researchers compared the DHEA levels of men with prostate cancer to those of healthy men. The prostate cancer patients (*Cancer Epidemiology Biomarkers* v 2, 1993) had 12 percent lower DHEA levels than the healthy men. Other studies have shown that, in general, higher DHEA levels can help prevent prostate disease. It also helps cure it as well.

At the University of Vienna (*Prostate* v 44, 2000), men with prostate cancer were compared to healthy controls. The doctors found the same results.

At the Urologische Klinik in Budapest (*Magyar Onkologia* v 14, 1970) over forty years ago, doctors studied prostate cancer patients and found that the men had low levels of DHEA. They suggested that such patients be treated with DHEA to normalize their levels.

At the Institute of Endocrinology in Berlin (*Experimental and Clinical Endocrinology Diabetes* v 99, 1992) doctors found, "DHEA levels in patients with prostate cancer were significantly lower."

At Huddinge University in Sweden (*Prostate* v 13, 1988), doctors performed an in-depth study, involving ten different hormones of seventy-eight men with prostate cancer. The research showed that men with high, youthful levels of DHEA and DHEA-S had a much better prognostic outlook, especially with regards to whether the cancer spread and metastasized. This excellent study included twenty-two references. Whether the cancer metastasizes is critical to the length and quality of life.

Dosage

You can take 25 mg of DHEA daily if you prove to be low by saliva or blood testing.

You should retest your levels annually to make sure your dose is proper and you are not aromatizing this into estrogens.

MELATONIN

In 1958, melatonin was identified as the pineal gland hormone, but it wasn't until the mid-1990s that it became available as an inexpensive supplement. There has been extensive research done on the prostate health benefits of melatonin, yet we never hear about any of this. The hallmark of this research is the discovery that the prostate actually contains melatonin receptors. Yet, medical doctors, including urologists, are not aware of this fact, and none of the prostate health books discuss melatonin. Figure 8.2, *Melatonin Levels Throughout Life,* shows that melatonin peaks around age thirteen, and then falls severely until it almost disappears around age sixty.

At the University of Lodz in Poland (*Neuroendocrine Letters* v 20, 1999), doctors showed that melatonin has beneficial effects on cancer in general. They said, "Melatonin may exert its oncostatic (cancer defeating) effect indirectly, via modulation of

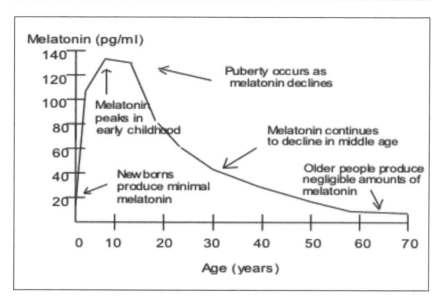

Figure 8.2. Melatonin Levels Throughout Life. This figure illustrates how melatonin levels fall as you age. Melantonin levels tend to peak around age thirteen. After that, the amount of melatonin in our bodies falls steadily, and by the time we are sixty, we have little melatonin left.

the endocrine and immune systems." Other researchers at the University of Lodz (*International Journal of Thymology* v 4, 1996) came to the same conclusion, that melatonin should be used as a standard means of treating prostate cancer. "Moreover," they stated, "preliminary results of use of melatonin in the treatment of cancer patients suggest possible therapeutic role for melatonin in human malignancy." Why isn't melatonin supplementation used as a standard cancer therapy now?

At the San Gerardo Hospital in Milan (*Prostate* v 45, 2000) researchers discovered dramatic benefits after giving melatonin to men with prostate cancer. Doctors reported (*Journal of Pineal Research* v 2, 1985) that men with BPH and prostate cancer had low melatonin levels, and that melatonin therapy should be used for these conditions. Doctors in China (*Zhongguo Yaolixue Tongbao* v 24, 2008) published a heavily referenced review on the melatonin studies, They concluded, "Melatonin is a promising agent for cancer treatment and prevention." Researchers at the University of Hong Kong (the *Journal of Pineal Research* v 43, 2007) also called for, "the use of melatonin in prostate cancer prevention" as standard therapy.

As a result of all the impressive animal studies, scientists have also conducted human studies on the benefits of melatonin. At the University of Tübingen in Germany (*Clinica Chimica Acta* v 209, 1992), researchers realized that men with both BPH and prostate cancer had low melatonin levels. In a later study at the same university (*Wiener Klinische Wochenschrift* v 109, 1997), doctors observed the same phenomenon in men with prostate cancer. The doctors suggested that using melatonin supplements to treat prostate cancer should be standard therapy.

A third study (*7th Colloquium of the European Pineal Society,* 1996) found low levels of melatonin in prostate cancer patients. A fourth study (*International Congressional Series,* 1993) strongly recommended giving melatonin to all men with prostate cancer as standard therapy. Other researchers at the University of Tübingen composed a long review of prostate cancer studies (*Advances in Experimental and Medical Biology* v 467, 1999) that included seventy-one references. All of them consistently showed that breast and prostate cancer patients have low levels of melatonin. They recommended using melatonin as standard therapy. The sixth study (*Neuroendocrine Letters* v 5, 1983) emphasized the "dynamic" effect of melatonin on prostate cancer growth. Men with both BPH and prostate cancer were found to have low melatonin levels.

For years, medical doctors and researchers all over the world have been recommending melatonin supplements as a standard treatment for prostate cancer. The mainstream media refuses to report this, so the general public doesn't know how beneficial melatonin really is.

The only way to test your levels is with a saliva test kit at 3 A.M. Do a Google search.

Dosage

Take melatonin supplements only at night, after the sun goes down, never during the day. Research has shown that taking 3 mg a night is a safe and effective dose. The media damned melatonin with faint praise as a mere sleep aid. In fact, it is a powerful and proven anti-aging, anti-cancer antioxidant that stimulates the immune system. Melatonin is a very powerful hormone!

PREGNENOLONE

Pregnenolone is the "grandmother" hormone from which all other sex steroid hormones are derived. It is most important as a brain metabolism regulator, and is largely responsible for memory, learning, and cognition. Pregnenolone might be called the forgotten hormone, as very little research has been done on its role in the endocrine system. It is the most potent memory enhancer known to science. Yet, endocrinologists and urologists are basically unaware of how important it is to measure and supplement pregnenolone, especially in people over the age of forty. Why has there been so little research on such a basic and powerful hormone?

As Figure 8.3 shows, pregnenolone falls precipitously after the age of thirty-five. No saliva testing kits for pregnenolone are currently available. There is no reason to use a doctor, when you can use inexpensive online blood testing labs without one. Almost no research has been done on pregnenolone and prostate health in the last three decades. Since our hormones work together as a team, common sense tell you to balance your pregnenolone levels.

Fortunately, at the famous Marie Curie Hospital in Paris (*Journal of Steroid Chemistry and Molecular Biology* v 46, 1993) doctors carried out an extensive, unusually sophisticated, and very detailed study on pregnenolone. They measured the levels of fourteen different hormones in men with prostate cancer and

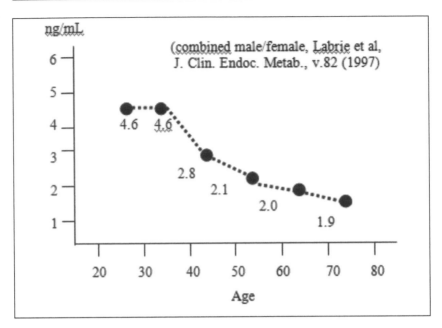

Figure 8.3. Pregnenolone Levels Throughout Life. This figure indicates how our pregnenolone levels fall as the body ages. Note that pregnenolone levels drop quickly starting around the age of thirty-five, and are usually only half what they were at their peak by the age of forty-five.

compared them to the hormone levels of healthy men. They discovered that pregnenolone (and DHEA) levels were generally lower in the prostate cancer patients.

Dosage

A good dose of pregnenolone for those over forty is 50 mg a day for men and 25 mg a day for women. Do not exceed these doses.

HUMAN GROWTH HORMONE

Human growth hormone (HGH) levels fall as we age. Raising your HGH levels only has modest benefits. At the University of Naples Federico II in Italy (*Journal of Clinical Endocrinology & Metabolism* v 88, 2003), a case-control study was done on the effects of falling HGH levels on prostate health. Researchers stated, "In conclusion, GH replacement restores prostate size to normal in both young and elderly patients with no increase in prostate abnormalities."

Real human growth hormone (rHGH) costs about $2,400 a year, and must be injected subcutaneously (under the skin). It is sold freeze dried. Once it is reconstituted and refrigerated, it goes bad in only one week. If you shock it or shake it, the 191 amino acid chain breaks, and it is useless. It is not some "miracle hormone" by any means, despite the media hype. It is expensive only because the pharmaceutical corporations have colluded to make it so. Veterinary growth hormones for farmers are very inexpensive and also have a 191 amino acid chain.

There are many products on the market that purport to raise HGH levels. *None of them have any value at all.* None of them work, no matter how well the ads are written. The jellyfish product has no value. You can maintain a youthful level of the human growth hormone by eating a low-calorie whole grain based diet, exercising regularly, taking proven supplements, balancing your other hormones, not using prescription or recreational drugs, fasting, and avoiding bad habits like smoking. HGH levels must be measured by multiple blood draws over a twelve hour period in a lab. People over fifty can be sure their levels are low. Go by the real world *results* you get. The money and effort spent will simply not equal the modest results you get.

Insulin like growth factor-1 (IGF-1) levels do not parallel HGH levels, despite the conventional wisdom. High IGF-1 levels are often associated with prostate disease. Don't even consider HGH unless you are over fifty and all your other basic hormones are balanced.

Dosage

HGH is very overrated because it is expensive. Only those over fifty, who have balanced all their other basic hormones, should even consider using HGH. You can support your HGH levels by taking one g of L-glutamine in the A.M. and one g in the P.M., daily. This may not work over the long term, though.

TRIIODOTHYRONINE AND THYROXINE

Prostate disease is often associated with thyroid dysfunction (*Journal of Urology* v 168, 2002 and *Prostate Cancer* v 4, 2001). You should test both your free, unbound T3 and T4 levels. You must be midrange, and not merely in range. If the range is, say, 2 to 8, you must be about 5. Remember, all of our hormones work together, in concert, as a unified system. You should test your free triiodothyronine (T3) and free L-thyroxine (T4) instead of your thyroid stimulating hormone (TSH) and T3 uptake, as your doctor might suggest. There are now blood spot tests for free T3 and free T4, but no saliva tests. You can also use Internet labs without a doctor.

Dosage

You should only take T3 and T4 supplements if you have a thyroid deficiency. Pharmaceutical T4 (Synthroid, Levoxyl, etc.) and T3 (Tiromel, etc.) are bioidentical in every way. Treat your T3 and T4 levels completely separately, and do not use Armour Thyroid® unless both your T3 and T4 levels are equally low. Armour® pig extract contains both T3 and T4 in a four to one ratio. It can only be used by about 5 percent of those who are hypothyroid.

INSULIN

High insulin levels have been positively correlated with BPH as well as cancer (the *Journal of Urology* v 168, 2002, *Recent Results in Cancer Research* v 166, 2005, and the *Journal of the National Cancer Institute* v 95, 2003). Most Americans have a blood insulin level of about 8 to 9 mIU/ml, when it should be only 4 to 5. The average Japanese level is under 5.

Insulin resistance is another cause of prostate disease

(*Hormone and Metabolic Research* v 35, 2003) which occurs when your body's cells cannot properly respond when insulin tries to transport glucose from the bloodstream into the muscle tissues. The only way you can diagnose this is by taking a glucose tolerance test (GTT). You simply drink a small cup of glucose solution, wait one hour, and test your blood sugar level. A GTT is an inexpensive test that everyone over forty should take. Your GTT result should be twenty points below the official medical accepted level.

Your fasting blood glucose should be 85 or less (not 100 or less). Insulin resistance (and diabetes) can be cured with a whole grain-based diet that avoids sugars, including honey, fruit, and fruit juice as much as possible. Add proper supplements, hormone balancing, exercise, no prescription drugs, or bad habits. You may not be able to fast until you are well. You can get an HbA1c kit at drugstores inexpensively. You want a level of 4.7, and not the medically accepted level of 6.5 mg/L. Remember that 4.7 number.

Dosage

As long as you maintain a healthy, low-sugar, low-fat, low-calorie whole grain-based diet, your blood sugar and insulin will normalize. Read my book *The Natural Diabetes Cure*.

CORTISOL

Cortisol is produced by the adrenal gland, and it is released when the body responds to stress; its primary functions are to suppress the immune system, increase blood sugar, and regulate the metabolism. Cortisol can only be measured with a series of four saliva tests, since levels vary so much during the day. You could do this by measuring levels at 9:00 A.M., 1:00 P.M., 5:00 P.M., and 9:00 P.M. All this really isn't worth the time and trouble. As you change your diet and lifestyle, and balance your other hormones, your cortisol levels will tend to normalize.

CONCLUSION

The hormones discussed throughout this chapter are all necessary in order for your body to function optimally. It is particularly important for men with prostate disease to maintain
healthy hormone levels. While androgens like testosterone and
DHEA are especially vital to prostate health, each of the basic
hormones provides dramatic health benefits to your prostate.
It's a good idea to test your hormone levels annually, so that
you can maintain a healthy hormone balance. All our hormones
work together in harmony as a concert. All illnesses are due in
part to hormone imbalance. This is simple, easy, inexpensive,
and no doctor is required.

9. Testosterone Is Your Friend

Nearly every medical doctor and urologist in the world will tell you that testosterone is bad for your prostate, and makes prostate cancer grow. This has become an unquestionable sacred dogma for doctors, but is 180 degrees opposed to reality. The fall in testosterone, as men age, almost exactly parallels the rise in prostatitis, BPH, and prostate cancer.

This insanity began more than eighty years ago, even before Charles Huggins got the brilliant idea to use castration as a cure for prostate cancer! This is prima facie insanity. Men with prostate cancer who get chemically castrated get very sickly from lack of testosterone and soon die. The damage from castration is obviously catastrophic, just as castration for women (hysterectomy) is equally catastrophic. This butchery has continued, but now doctors use chemicals ("ablation") to castrate men instead of scalpels.

There are over 200 published studies in our files from clinics around the world proving beyond any doubt that *testosterone helps prevent and cure all forms of prostate disease.* In this chapter, there are thirty-one published studies that prove empirically that testosterone is prostate healthy. Every year more such studies are published, yet doctors still chemically castrate men in order to reduce their testosterone levels to zero. In 2016, some doctors finally started giving testosterone supplementation to prostate cancer patients with dramatic results.

THE HISTORY OF TESTOSTERONE

A study on testosterone from Oxford University was published in the *Proceedings of the Royal Society of Medicine* in 1936. Testosterone was only discovered and synthesized in 1935, so it was barely known to doctors, much less available. Ironically, even eighty years ago, doctors knew that estrogen was bad for prostate health, and testosterone was good for prostate health. They also were aware of the all-important testosterone-to-estrogen ratio, in which testosterone should control and limit the "female hormone."

Another study from Louisiana State University was published in the *Journal of Urology* in 1938. In this case, the doctors understood that testosterone levels fall as men age, and the incidence of prostate disease rises greatly. Doctors gave patients testosterone (from animal testes) with good results. The medical profession inherently knew that "the male hormone" was good for curing BPH, a common malady even then.

THE SCIENCE BEHIND TESTOSTERONE

As you can clearly see from Figure 9.1, *Male Estrogen and Testosterone Blood Levels Throughout Life*, testosterone levels fall as men age, while estrogen levels rise. Testosterone dominance and the testosterone-to-estrogen ratio are reversed. The probability of developing prostate disease increases accordingly. Remember, common sense tells you that testosterone is your friend, has always been your friend, and will always be your friend.

The scientific literature is full of countless studies that prove testosterone is necessary for a healthy prostate and metabolism. When free testosterone levels in the blood are low, the prostate receptors must choose dihydrotestosterone (DHT) instead. DHT binding to the prostate is a basic cause of illness. High serum

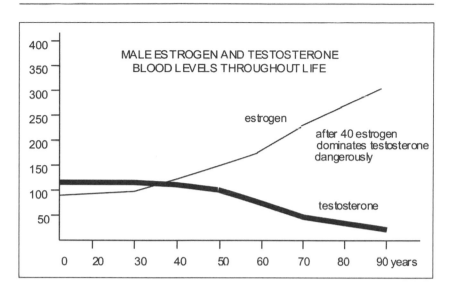

Figure 9.1. Male Estrogen and Testosterone Blood Levels Throughout Life.
This figure depicts the average man's estrogen and testosterone levels
throughout his life. Note that during his youth, a man's testosterone
levels will be higher than his estrogen levels. But after he turns thirty,
his testosterone-to-estrogen ratio begins to reverse, and estrogen
dominates testosterone; this reversal is very dangerous to men's health.
Adapted from *Acta Endrocrinologica* v 74, 1973 and v 80, 1970.

DHT can be harmful to prostate health. Let's take just some of
the many dozens of published clinical studies from around the
world to prove that high, youthful levels of the androgens testosterone, androstenedione, and DHEA protect you from prostate illness. Supplementing low testosterone and DHEA levels
will help cure your illness. Every month, more such studies are
published in the international medical literature.

A progressive, innovative, and pioneering doctor named
Richmond Prehn, at the University of Washington[1], published a
stunning article in 1999. He said that we should consider using
androgen *supplementation* to reduce the growth of prostate cancer! He pointed out that declining testosterone levels contribute
to carcinogenesis, and that supplementing low levels would
reduce cancer rates. He referred to earlier studies that showed
low testosterone levels in prostate cancer patients indicated a

much worse prognosis. It is doctors like him that are going to lead us into the medical Age of Enlightenment, and out of the Age of Darkness.

At the University of Witwaterstrand[2] in South Africa, researchers conducted a study, *Low Serum Testosterone Predicts a Poor Outcome in Meta-static Prostate Cancer.* They studied 122 patients, and found that the ones with the *highest* testosterone levels had the least aggressive tumors, and lived the longest. The patients with the lowest testosterone levels had far more aggressive growths, and died much sooner. The doctors concluded, "Low testosterone seems to result in a more aggressive disease and a poorer prognosis in advanced prostate cancer." This study is very clear.

At the Hubei Medical University in China[3], doctors studied men with BPH and carcinoma and discovered, "The results showed that serum testosterone in patients with BPH and prostate cancer antigens (PCA) was lower than that of the healthy control group." Further, ". . . the ratio of testosterone-to-estradiol is decreased with the rise of the age. The results suggested that the imbalance of serum sex hormones (i.e., falling testosterone and rising estrogen) was related to the pathogenesis of BPH and PCA." *It is low testosterone and high estrogen levels that cause prostate problems.*

At Harvard Medical School[4], doctors carried out a study titled *Is Low Serum Testosterone a Marker for High Grade Prostate Cancer?* They found the men with lower testosterone levels had more aggressive tumors, higher Gleason scores (a measure of cancer severity), and shorter life spans. The conclusion: "In our study, patients with prostate cancer and low free testosterone had more extensive disease. In addition, all men with a biopsy Gleason score of 8 or greater had low serum free testosterone. This finding suggests that low serum free testosterone may be a marker for more aggressive disease." Again, the lower the testosterone, the worse the prognosis. Directly from Harvard Medical School.

At the University of Vienna[5], men with prostate cancer were studied for their serum testosterone levels. The doctors concluded, "Low serum testosterone in men with newly diagnosed prostate cancer is associated with higher tumor microvessel and androgen receptor density (both of these promote malignancies), as well as higher Gleason score, suggesting enhanced malignant potential." In men with low testosterone, the tumors grew faster, the cancer was more aggressive, and the patients died sooner.

Another study from the University of Vienna[6] was titled, *High Grade Prostate Cancer is Associated With Low Serum Testosterone Levels*. These researchers found that "patients with high Gleason score prostate cancer have lower testosterone levels." The men with the lowest Gleason scores and slowest growing malignancies had high testosterone levels. Those with the highest Gleason scores and fastest growing malignancies had low testosterone levels.

Another study at Harvard[7] found that the cancer patients with the highest levels of testosterone fared the best, and lived the longest: "A high prevalence of biopsy detectable prostate cancer was identified in men with low total or free testosterone."

Doctors at the Memphis Veterans Administration Hospital[8] discovered that elderly veterans fared much better when they had higher testosterone levels. They stated, "Patients with a pretreatment testosterone level of less than 300 ng/100 ml had shorter intervals free of progression than patients with pretreatment testosterone levels of greater than 300 ng/100 ml." The doctors referred to studies conducted as early as 1971 that showed the same previous phenomenon. The higher their testosterone levels, the longer the men lived; the lower their levels, the sooner they died.

In an impressive collective effort between six international clinics, scientists used the Norwegian Cancer Registry to study the frozen blood serum and medical records of approximately 28,000 men with an average age of sixty. The scientists found that the healthy men actually had higher testosterone levels than the ones who developed prostate cancer. They concluded low testosterone increases prostate cancer rates. Men, this study is the second largest ever done on testosterone and prostate cancer. *You just can't argue with their conclusions based on 28,000 real men.*

The University of Chicago[10] found the exact same results. "A separate analysis of serum testosterone levels revealed that the higher the pretreatment serum testosterone level, the greater the survival rate." The higher the testosterone levels were, the longer the men lived, and the better they fared. Doctors should be giving men testosterone therapy, rather than androgen ablation.

At Johns Hopkins University in Baltimore[11], three groups of men were studied: healthy, BPH, and cancer. Their testosterone was measured over a five-year period. The healthy men had an average level of 636.1 (ng/ml), the BPH group only 527.4, and the men with localized cancer averaged only 472.6. Clearly, the healthy men had much higher levels of testosterone.

At the University of Utah[12], researchers carried out a unique study of 214 sets of male twins. Using identical twins is a most effective means to demonstrate scientific validity. The researchers found that "Prostate volumes correlated inversely with age-adjusted serum testosterone." The higher the testosterone levels, the smaller the men's prostate glands were—proof that you need youthful testosterone levels for good prostate health.

At the Petrov Institute in Russia[13], middle aged men were given testosterone. Their prostates reduced in volume, generally in six months. "These findings suggest that exogenous testosterone in middle-aged and older men with some clinical features of age-related androgen deficiency can retard or reverse prostate growth." Everyone knows that the gradual decrease in male testosterone levels after the age of thirty clearly coincides with the abnormal increase in prostate volumes. The need for testosterone supplementation is obvious, yet doctors somehow can't see this.

At the famous Tenovus Institute in Wales[14], over 200 prostate cancer patients were studied. Again, doctors found that the men with the lowest testosterone levels had the poorest prognosis and died the soonest. "Low concentrations of testosterone at the time of diagnosis related to a poor prognosis. Patients who died within one year of diagnosis had the lowest mean levels of this steroid." They went on to repeat, "The results of this study suggest that low testosterone concentrations in men with prostatic carcinoma at the time of initial diagnosis is associated with a poor prognosis. The highest levels of testosterone were found in those patients who subsequently survived the longest." This study was done over thirty years ago, and was published in a major medical journal. Why are doctors still ignorant of all this?

Doctors at Baylor University[15] finally came out and said, "Given this physiological concept, many clinical investigators have begun to promote testosterone supplementation therapy as safe in men with prostate cancer." The study was titled *Testosterone Therapy in Men with Prostate Cancer*, with a full fifty-one references.

Abraham Morgantaler at Harvard[16] has been the leading proponent of giving prostate cancer patients testosterone therapy. "There is not now—nor has there ever been—a scientific basis for the belief that testosterone causes prostate cancer to grow." He went on to say, "The assertion that higher testosterone enhances prostate cancer growth has persisted as a medical myth since 1941, despite all evidence to the contrary." In the same journal eight years later, he said, "It may therefore be reasonable to consider testosterone therapy in men with prostate cancer and hypogonadism." He has published numerous other studies stating this. Congratulations!

In 1978, at the Granada Medical Facility[17], men with BPH were studied and compared with healthy men. The men with BPH had a 43 percent lower testosterone level than the healthy men. Researchers stated that "the testosterone concentration in the BPH group was significantly lower (43%) than that of the healthy control group." They proved it is excess estradiol and estrone that cause prostate disease. This study was published over thirty years ago in a major medical journal, yet is still ignored today.

At the Royal London Hospital[18] doctors conducted a stunning review of thirty-four studies, complete with fifty-five references. They revealed that the Huggins testosterone dogma has been completely unsupported by science for the last sixty years, "yet there has so far been no conclusive evidence, despite thirty-four studies, that levels of circulating testosterone in individuals developing prostate cancer are higher than in controls." They went on to say, "Firstly, prostate cancers arising in men with low serum testosterone levels are more malignant and frequently unresponsive to hormones (e.g. estrogen)." Yet most all doctors continue to walk in darkness.

At the Beth Israel Hospital in New York City[19], researchers studied men for thirteen different hormones to determine which ones contributed to the growth of their carcinomas. They found that the average cancer patient had a low testosterone level of about 350 ng/dl, compared to the healthy controls' much higher levels of about 450 ng/dl. In men under sixty-five, the difference was much more dramatic, with levels of 282 ng/dl in cancer patients compared to 434 ng/dl for the healthy controls—over 50 percent higher testosterone levels in healthy men without cancer. These researchers were very reluctant to admit what they found, however, because it contradicted their dogma.

In 2014, the University of California[20] and six other clinics published *Testosterone Replacement Therapy Following the Diagnosis of Prostate Cancer*. The title says it all. Here the doctors studied the medical records of 149,354 men. They ultimately stated that testosterone replacement therapy is a viable option for men with a history of prostate cancer. You have to realize how much courage it takes to make a statement like that. The next year, the same journal published a second study titled *Testosterone Replacement Therapy in Men with Prostate Cancer*, which verified their findings.

Thirty years ago, at the University of Helsinki[21], hormones were measured in men with BPH and prostate cancer, against healthy controls. The free testosterone levels of the BPH patients averaged only 301 pmol/L, the cancer patients just 249 pmol/L, while the healthy men had a high level of 380 pmol/L. The healthy men had low estradiol levels of only 53.5 pmol/L, while the BPH patients had a stunning 137.4 pmol/L, and the cancer patients 83.7 pmol/L. Furthermore, the healthy men had testosterone-to-estradiol ratios of 7.1:1 (the higher, the better), while the BPH men had 2.2:1, and the cancer patients 3.0:1. Yet the poor doctors still couldn't figure out that excess estrogens cause prostate disease, while high, youthful testosterone levels prevent and cure it. None so blind as those who will not see.

At Umea University Hospital in Sweden[22], almost 3,000 men, both with and without prostate cancer, were studied for their blood androgen levels. The men with the highest levels of testosterone had the least rates of cancer, while the men with the lowest levels of testosterone had the highest rates of cancer. The doctors were stunned at the results, since they clearly started out to prove that "androgens stimulate prostate cancer in vivo and in vitro." They began with a bias against testosterone, but had to reverse themselves due to their own findings.

In another study at Harvard Medical School[23] doctors really took a big risk in going against the prevailing negative view of testosterone and prostate health. They took seventy-five men with low testosterone, twenty of whom had a precancerous condition called "prostatic intraepithelial neoplasia" (PIN). They gave all of these men supplemental testosterone for one year, knowing that the prevailing medical opinion anticipates that those men with PIN will get outright cancer. Of course, nothing of the sort happened. The men were in much better mental and physical health after raising their testosterone levels. Their prostate glands prospered by having the testosterone they needed. These doctors deserve a lot of credit for their courage.

At Taipei Veterans Hospital[24], ninety-six men with advanced metastatic prostate cancer were studied for their hormone levels. The men were divided into two groups based on their testosterone levels. The group with 77 percent higher testosterone levels fared the best, lived the longest, and had the slowest tumor growth. The doctors concluded, "Higher testosterone and lower LH, FSH and prolactin levels were good prognostic factors for patients with metastatic prostate cancer irrespective of tumor grading." In the same journal, in the same year, another study *Circulating Free Testosterone is an Independent Predictor of Advanced Prostate Cancer* was published. This verified the results of the first study.

At the University of Perugia[25], doctors published *Low Serum Testosterone Levels are Predictive of Prostate Cancer*, with the assertion that "testosterone levels are predictive of prostate cancer, and that prostate cancer is frequently associated with low testosterone levels." Couldn't be clearer.

At Yamagata University in Japan[26] a first-rate study was carried out on men suffering from BPH. The men with BPH lower testosterone levels and higher estradiol levels compared to healthy controls. The healthy men had 49 percent higher free testosterone levels. The healthy men also had excellent testosterone-to-estrogen ratios.

At the Harvard School of Public Health and other clinics[27], elderly men with prostate cancer were compared to healthy men. The healthy controls had much higher testosterone levels than the cancer patients. This was a very powerful human "case-control study."

At Helsinki University in Finland,[28] 123 elderly men with prostate cancer were studied for their hormone levels. The researchers concluded, "Low pretreatment testosterone values indicated poorer prognosis." The lower the free testosterone levels, the higher the Gleason score. The lower the free testosterone, the more aggressive were the tumors. The lower the free testosterone, the more the cancer metastasized. The lower the free testosterone the sooner they died. After four years, 80 percent of the men with the higher testosterone levels were still alive, but only 45 percent of the men with the lower testosterone levels survived. High testosterone levels win again.

At the University of British Columbia *Testosterone Therapy in Patients with Treated and Untreated Prostate Cancer*[29] was published. Yes, they gave testosterone to prostate cancer patients. "Our study supports the hypothesis that testosterone therapy may be oncologically safe in hypogonadal men." Congratulations to these brave doctors. Modern urologists are now able to give their prostate cancer patients testosterone supplements without fear of losing their license, or being sued.

CONCLUSION

We could go on with dozens more studies on the benefits of testosterone, but thirty-one should be enough to show just how strong and comprehensive the evidence behind testosterone really is. Every year, researchers around the world conduct further studies, proving again and again that testosterone is not only beneficial, but also necessary for a healthy prostate. Soon, testosterone supplementation for prostate disease will be standard medical practice.

10. Estrogens

Men and women have exactly the same hormones, only in different amounts. There is no "estrogen," per se. The term estrogen is merely convenient to use when referring to the class of hormones collectively known as *estrogens*. Men have smaller amounts of estrogen than women until the age of fifty, when male levels begin to rise. Female levels fall after menopause. *So, middle-aged men commonly have more estrogen than women!*

As men's testosterone-to-estrogen ratios become reversed, the changes in their hormone levels can have very dangerous effects on their health. The reversal of this ratio is a major key to understanding not only prostate disease, but many other male illnesses, including cardiovascular health, diabetes, liver disease, low immunity, gynecomastia (male breast growth), obesity, baldness, and various cancers.

THE TRUTH ABOUT ESTROGENS

There are actually three basic estrogens: estradiol or E2 (the most powerful and most carcinogenic); estrone or E1; and estriol or E3 (the weakest, safest, and most beneficial estrogen). Estradiol and estrone comprise about 20 percent of human estrogen, and estriol about 80 percent. (Men rarely have any estriol imbalance, and do not need to test their estriol levels as women do.) The testosterone-to-estrogen ratio reversal that occurs as we age creates high levels of estradiol and estrone in men. High estradiol and estrone levels are a basic hormonal cause of prostate disease.

THE SCIENCE BEHIND
THE TESTOSTERONE-TO-ESTROGEN RATIO

Over the last fifty years there have been dozens of studies showing the harmful effect of excessive estrogen in aging males caused by the reversed androgen-to-estrogen ratio (including androstenedione and DHEA). We will pick twenty of them to quickly prove that testosterone is your friend, and excess estrogen is your enemy. The reversal of the androgen-to-estrogen ratio is the most important hormonal insight we have into prostate disease.

At the University of Hamburg (*Prostate* v 3, 1982), doctors found high levels of estrogens in men with prostate enlargement. "In conclusion, there is a distinct accumulation of estrogens in the nuclei of stroma, estradiol concentration being significantly higher—thus stimulating the growth of BPH." *Excessive estradiol and estrone are the main biochemical cause of prostate disease.* In a second study, performed at the same university (*Journal of Steroid Biochemistry* v 19, 1983), men with BPH were found to have excessive estradiol in their prostates, high 5-alpha-reductase activity, and increased DHT accumulation.

At the Bielanski Hospital in Poland (*Roczniki Akademii Medicina* v 42, 1984), men with prostate cancer generally had high serum estradiol and low serum testosterone, displaying the classic testosterone-to-estrogen ratio reversal. At the American Health Foundation in New York (*Prostate* v 5, 1984), doctors discovered that "persons with prostate cancer had higher estrone and estradiol levels in prostatic fluid."

At TNB College in India (*Indian Journal of Physiology and Pharmacology* v 29, 1985) scientists studied men with BPH. They found that the patients had high estrone levels in their prostate glands, but low pregnenolone levels. At the Sloan-Kettering Institute (*Prostate* v 9, 1986), researchers found high levels of estrogens in BPH patients: "Total estrogens produced in BPH patients was 223 fmol/mg compared with healthy controls with only 102 fmol/mg." Likewise, at the University of Miami (*Prostate* v 21, 1992) doctors found high estrogens in men with BPH; they concluded that "local estrogen production in the stroma and/or epithelium of the prostate plays a role in the . . . development of BPH."

Doctors at Schering AG in Berlin (*Journal of Steroid Biochemistry and Molecular Biology* v 44, 1993) recommended, "Consequently, estrogen deprivation might be a new, useful principle for a conservative treatment of BPH." At Ruhr University Bochum in Germany (*Journal of Clinical Endocrinology and Metabolism* v 77, 1993), doctors said, " . . . the prostatic accumulation of DHT, estradiol, and estrone is intimately correlated with aging, leading to the increase of the estrogen/testosterone ratio in BPH." Like their colleagues from other studies, these doctors also found higher estradiol and estrone levels in the glands of their BPH patients.

At the University of Bonn (*Journal of Steroid Biochemistry and Molecular Biology* v 44, 1993), doctors used estrogen blockers to lower estradiol and estrone in BPH patients with dramatic results. Serum estrogen levels fell strongly. Prostate volumes fell from 74.2 to 64.0 in only ninety days. The doctors strongly recommended estrogen deprivation for BPH. The problem here is that all prescription estrogen blockers are toxic, have serious side effects, and should not be used. *You can lower estradiol and estrone naturally with diet and lifestyle.* At Harvard Medical School (*Journal of Clinical Endocrinology* v 77, 1993), 320 men with BPH were compared to 320 healthy men. High plasma estradiol and low androgens were clearly related to BPH, as well as to the obviously reversed testosterone-to-estrogen ratio. Studies like these are groundbreaking, even though they took place over thirty years ago, yet are ignored today.

At Gunma University in Japan (*Scandinavian Journal of Urology and Nephrology* v 29, 1995), doctors stated that " . . . an estrogen dominated environment plays an important role in the development of BPH." Specifically, they determined that estrogen levels unmistakably and clearly correlated to prostate volumes.

At the University of Vienna (*Wiener Klinische Woschenschrift* v 110, 1998), twenty-three clinical trials, spanning fifteen years, were reviewed. The researchers found that estrogen (not testosterone) suppression was the proper treatment for BPH. "The estrogen suppression . . . is considered as an efficient pharmacotherapeutic strategy in the medical treatment of uncomplicated BPH." If these good doctors had reached a little further, they might have realized that testosterone supplementation is the next step.

In another study at Gunma University (*Prostate* v 42, 2000), doctors found high estradiol in BPH patients. A different group of doctors at Yamagata University came across similar results (*Journal of Urology* v 21, 2000): "Serum estradiol levels correlating with the prostate volume, whereas free testosterone levels did not." Still more Japanese doctors (*Rinsho Byori* v 52, 2004) determined, "Estrogen may play a pathophysiological role in BPH . . . . due to increased estrogen and decreased testosterone. Estrogen plays a physiological role in BPH." Back in the United States, the doctors at Northwestern University (*Prostate* v 41, 1999) came to the same conclusion. Estrogen dominates testosterone after a man reaches the age of fifty, and this hormonal trend is a major cause of prostate growth.

A 2007 review of the scientific literature (*Journal of Cellular Biochemistry* v 102) clearly indicated that high estrogen levels are the endocrinological cause of prostate disease. The researchers concluded, "Multiple, consistent evidence suggests that estrogens are critical players in human prostate cancer. Their role was only recently considered, being eclipsed for years by an androgen-dominated interest." Furthermore, a slightly more recent review (*European Journal of Cancer* v 44, 2008) stated, "This leads to the intriguing notion that estradiol may be the initiating driver of prostate cancer . . . anti-estrogens might be an over-looked treatment."

Another study published the very same year (*Journal of Steroid Biochemistry and Molecular Biology* v 109, 2008) found estrone to be "significantly higher in prostate cancer." Yet another study from 2008 (*Journal of Endocrinology* v 197, 2008) stated, "Estrogens have been implicated as a cause of BPH. These findings support the hypothesis that estrogen plays a role in the pathogenesis of BPH."

A recent study (the *European Journal of Cancer Prevention* v 19, 2010) found high estrogens in prostate cancer, stating that "the action of unopposed estrogen directly initiates, promotes, and exacerbates prostatic enlargement and prostate cancer. *This controversial breakthrough represents a paradigm shift in medical thinking, which can prevent the raging pandemic of cancer sweeping the world.*" The doctors also found unopposed estrogen to be the base cause of obesity, diabetes, and breast cancer. In a different study from 2010 (*Urology* v 76, 2010), the researchers clearly stated, "In this cohort of older men, higher estrone levels were strongly associated with increased risk of incident prostate cancer."

For decades, researchers and scientists have revealed the prostate health benefits of testosterone, along with the dangers of estrogens. Note that there is also overwhelming evidence from animal studies (which date back over fifty years) that proves that the estrogens estradiol and estrone are basic contributors to BPH, prostatitis, and cancer. These studies are so numerous you can't count them all. The worldwide clinical trials verify that high estrogen levels are a basic cause of all prostate disease, not androgens.

CONCLUSION

High estradiol and estrone levels are the real endocrine cause of prostate disease. Unfortunately, it is difficult to lower estrogen levels. The current prescription estrogen blockers and aromatase inhibitors are very toxic, dangerous, and have serious side effects. Aromatase is the enzyme that converts testosterone to estradiol, and androstenedione to estrone. It was only recently discovered, and not well understood at all. It is very difficult to lower aromatase, or to prevent aromatase activity. Diet and lifestyle only do so much here. It may be decades before we find safe, effective methods to lower aromatase activity.

Remember, you can only lower estrogen levels by eating a whole grain diet, not eating animal fats, consuming fewer calories, staying slim, avoiding alcohol and caffeine, and exercising regularly. You should also take DIM and flax oil to help lower your estradiol and estrone. It is especially important to avoid eating saturated animal fats. Consuming saturated animal fats and being overweight are the two biggest causes of elevated estradiol and estrone levels. The most important factor here is maintaining a low-fat diet by only consuming vegetable oils in moderation.

11. Home Hormone Testing

Prostate conditions are largely hormone-based. Our prostates are more affected by hormones than any other factor. Ironically, even urologists almost never test their patients' hormone levels, especially testosterone. If you were to demand a hormone test from your doctor, it would require getting blood drawn, paying up to $100 per hormone tested, going on a second office visit, and paying for expensive prescriptions. The test results that come back to you often do not distinguish between bound (unavailable levels) and free (bioavailable levels). Ranges can very vague, and not age-adjusted.

Most doctors do not know the difference between bound and unbound hormones. In fact, most doctors are simply unaware of which hormones to test, how to test them, and how to administer supplemental ones. Even urologists, endocrinologists, naturopaths, and holistic doctors are surprisingly uninformed about hormone testing and administration, though this is their specialty. This means it is left up to you to be your own doctor and test your hormone levels. Test your own levels with saliva kits, blood spot kits, and online Internet labs without a doctor.

UNDERSTANDING HOW HOME HORMONE TESTING WORKS

Proteins in our bloodstream called sex hormone-binding globulins (SHBG) bind themselves to the majority of our sex hormones, making them biologically unavailable. Testosterone, for example, is about 98 percent bound. This leaves only about 2 percent free, bioavailable testosterone that actually affects our metabolic processes. Only your free, unbound hormone levels matter.

For over thirty years now, scientists have been able to accurately measure hormone levels by using saliva and blood spot samples. Previously, this has taken place only in clinics and medical studies. Now, with technological advances, saliva and blood samples can be collected at home, and sent to a laboratory for a radioimmunoassay (RIA) analysis. All this can be achieved at a cost of only $35 per hormone.

The World Health Organization approved this method of hormone testing in the 1990s due to its ease, efficiency, reliability, and practicality. Now you can test estradiol, estrone, estriol, testosterone, DHEA, melatonin, T3, T4, and cortisol by simply sending your sample to a testing lab. Pregnenolone, progesterone, and insulin must be tested with blood draws. Some states, including California, Maryland, and New York, ban home hormone testing in order to protect the medical profession's monopoly. That is criminal!

Saliva and blood spot testing is a tremendous breakthrough in both traditional medicine and alternative, natural medicine. Very few people are aware of it, and even fewer know where to buy the test kits. You would think these kits would be available in every pharmacy and drugstore. It may take years for such a great advance in diagnostic medicine to become widely utilized. You can also find online labs that test your hormones without a doctor. They refer you to a clinic in your city for a real, and inexpensive, blood draw. Healthcheckusa.com is one popular online lab testing website.

MEASURING AND BALANCING
THE LEVELS OF YOUR BASIC HORMONES

No matter what illness you are suffering from, remember that doctors of any kind rarely test your basic hormones. Basically, men (and women) would test testosterone, DHEA, estradiol, estrone, T3, T4, and insulin. Women would add estriol. Your hormones are critical to every aspect of your health, including mental functioning. Young people who are ill should have their basic hormones tested. Everyone over the age of forty definitely needs to test their levels. You will never enjoy good health and long life unless your endocrine system is balanced at youthful levels.

It is not well known that men and women have exactly the same hormones, only in different amounts. Women have the androgens DHEA, testosterone, and androstenedione. Men have progesterone, prolactin (the milk secreting hormone), luteinizing hormone (LH), follicle-stimulating hormone (FSH), and the three basic estrogens. Women even have a prostate specific antigen (PSA), yet they have no prostate gland! The vast majority of people have no idea what any of their vital hormone levels are, or whether they are too high or too low. You can never know the true state of your health, or obtain your optimum health, unless you know your basic hormone levels and balance them to youthful ranges. It would be ideal to achieve the levels you had at age thirty. Youthful levels are your goal.

Testosterone

Over 90 percent of men over the age of fifty have low testosterone and need supplementation. Refer to Figure 11.1, *Salivary Testosterone Levels Throughout Life,* to see how testosterone levels in our saliva fall significantly as we age. Measure your free (not bound) testosterone. You can improve your testosterone levels by using a half gram of a 3 percent transdermal cream. However, 80 percent is wasted this way. Or you can take 4 mg of a sublingual testosterone salt (such as enathate) in vegetable oil (free base testosterone tastes terrible). This will give you 3 mg of actual testosterone.

You can make your own dimethyl sulfoxide (DMSO) solution and use 3 mg of free testosterone or 4 mg of testosterone

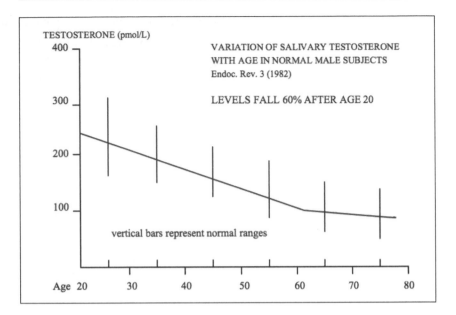

Figure 11.1 Salivary Testosterone Levels Throughout Life. This chart illustrates how your salivary testosterone levels fall as you age. By measuring your testosterone levels with saliva test kits, you can determine whether or not you need a testosterone supplement. Testosterone levels peak around age twenty, but fall 60 percent from then on. So, 90 percent of men over the age of fifty can and should benefit from proper testosterone supplements.

enanthate. Use on thin skin only, such as your inner wrists. Take your testosterone supplement only in the morning, and never use oral forms, injections, patches, implants, weak gels, or steroids.

Watch out for androgen resistance due to high aromatase activity. This condition will result in high estradiol and estrone levels, but low testosterone levels. If you suffer from high aromatase activity, there is simply no cure for this. You cannot use testosterone, androstenedione, pregnenolone, HCG, suicide aromatase inhibitors, or any pro- or pre-testosterone drug at all. It may be decades before we find out how to safely and effectively lower aromatase activity. This is genetic, so diet and lifestyle will only be of limited help.

Dehydroepiandrosterone

Measure your free DHEA or DHEA-S (sulfate) levels. Again, you want the youthful level you had at age thirty. If your levels are low, you can take 25 mg of oral DHEA. DHEA is called the "life extension hormone" for good reason. If your DHEA is too high, only diet and lifestyle will lower it. If taking DHEA causes a rise in estradiol or estrone, then you are androgen resistant and cannot take any androgen or pro-androgen supplement.

Estrogens

As discussed in the previous chapter, there are three major estrogens. As men age, their estradiol and estrone levels rise, while their testosterone level falls. This reverses the traditional testosterone-to-estrogen ratio, and causes serious problems, such as prostate disease, breast enlargement, baldness, weight gain, heart problems, and many other conditions. (Estriol is rarely out of line in men.)

Test your free (not bound) estradiol and estrone levels with a saliva test kit. *You want low normal levels* ideally, and you can use the postmenopausal female levels for your range. This test is very important, since these two estrogens are the basic internal cause of prostate disease. If your levels are normal, or higher, then lower them with diet and lifestyle. Do not use toxic prescription anti-aromatase or estrogen-blocker drugs.

Progesterone

We have seen already how important progesterone is. This should be measured by a serum (not plasma or saliva) blood draw, as it is fat-soluble. Actually, you really don't need to test your progesterone levels. Just use 1/8 teaspoon of a good transdermal cream five days a week. You can apply this to thin skin like that on your inner wrist, or directly to your scrotum for even better results. Progesterone is safe and nontoxic, so you don't have to worry about taking too much with a mere 1/8 teaspoon, and only five days a week at that.

Cortisol

Using a four sample (9/1/5/9) profile is the only realistic way to measure your cortisol levels. Cortisol levels vary greatly during the day and night. You really don't need to test your cortisol levels at all. Cortisol is what it is. Only diet and lifestyle will raise or lower your levels effectively. Diet and lifestyle will help normalize your levels.

Insulin and Blood Sugar

Insulin must be tested with an inexpensive blood draw. You can use online labs without a doctor. You want a level of 4 to 5 mIU/ml. Your fasting blood sugar level should be 85 or less. Remember that magic number—85 or less.

You should also get a one-hour glucose tolerance test (GTT) to determine possible insulin resistance. This tells you how your body reacts to sugar intake. Look for a result of 20 mg/dl less than the accepted standard.

You can also buy glycated hemoglobin (HbA1c) kits inexpensively at the drugstore; these give you a six-month average of your blood sugar levels. Look for a level of 4.7 to equate with a blood sugar level of 85. High blood sugar and insulin resistance is epidemic in America. Now we know these contribute to prostate disease, so keep your blood sugar and insulin low.

Human Growth Hormone

Human growth hormone (HGH) falls dramatically as we age. This is a very overrated and expensive hormone. It will cost $1,200 to $2,400 a year for one IU daily, and should be injected.

HGH levels vary radically during the day, especially when you are asleep. If you want to test your HGH levels, you must go to a specialty clinic and get a twelve-hour profile. IGF-1 levels do not parallel HGH levels, despite the common wisdom. In fact, men with prostate disease usually have high IGF-1 levels.

If you are over fifty, and want to use HGH, just go by actual physical, measurable benefits achieved after ninety days. As discussed earlier, diet and lifestyle will keep your HGH levels up. *None of the over-the-counter supplements have any legitimacy at all,* regardless of their impressive claims.

You must use real prescription HGH daily by injection. Sublingual use in DMSO also works, but doctors cannot prescribe this form. The molecule is too large to use with DMSO for regular transdermal use. The HGH molecule chain is very long (191 amino acids) and will not go through the skin intact. You cannot shake or shock HGH, or it will break and become useless.

The bottom line: HGH is overrated simply because it is very expensive. If you are over fifty, balance all your other hormones before even considering HGH therapy.

Melatonin

Melatonin has to be tested separately, as it must be collected by itself at 3:00 in the morning. If you are over forty, you can generally safely take 3 mg of melatonin at night without first testing your levels. A few companies do offer melatonin saliva kits, and it is obviously not realistic to go to a sleep clinic in the middle of the night to measure your melatonin levels.

Pregnenolone

In 2018, pregnenolone saliva testing kits are not available. If you are over forty, you can generally safely take 50 mg. Find an Internet blood testing service without a doctor. Soon we should have a wider choice in saliva test kits that include pregnenolone.

Triiodothyronine and Thyroxine

Low thyroid function is epidemic in Western countries, and doctors are especially poor in diagnosing this. Just get your free triiodothyronine (T3) and free thyroxine (T4) levels measured with a blood draw or blood spot kits. *These levels must be mid-range*, and not merely "in range". Low normal range is called "subclinical hypothyroidism." If the normal scale is, say, 6 to12, then you want to be as close to 9 as possible.

Doctors will generally tell you that you are fine if you are in range, but this is just not true. Your levels must be midrange for both free T3 and free T4. You don't need to be concerned with any other thyroid tests unless you have a serious problem with this gland. Use a blood spot kit, or one of the Internet blood testing services without a doctor. Web sites like healthcheckusa. com, for example, will test your hormone levels inexpensively, no doctor necessary.

CONCLUSION

Search the Internet for "saliva hormone testing" or "saliva hormone test" to find home hormone testing kits. For blood tests, just search for "online blood testing.". The saliva kits just aren't sold in retail stores yet. If you live outside of the United States, you can send in the saliva kits using couriers such as UPS. Always test your hormone samples around 9:00 A.M. (except melatonin) for consistency. You should monitor the levels of all your basic hormones (that you choose to supplement) at least once a year.

Balancing your hormone levels is one of the last steps along the way to a healthy prostate. Together with a whole grain-based diet, proven supplements, exercise, regular fasting, no bad habits, and no prescription drugs, hormone balancing will greatly improve your health. These seven steps are all you need to cure prostate disease.

Seven Steps
to Natural Health

The following steps are of vital importance if you want to live a long and healthy life. With these seven steps you can cure "incurable" illnesses like cancer, diabetes, and heart disease using natural treatments rather than dangerous prescription drugs, surgery, or chemotherapy. Do your best to follow every step, and note that there is also an optional eighth step that recommends prayer or meditation.

1. Eat an American macrobiotic whole grain-based diet. Diet is the most crucial factor in achieving good health. *Diet cures disease*. Everything else is secondary. Diet is everything.

2. Take proven supplements to enhance the effects of your diet. There are forty-seven scientifically recommended supplements for those over forty.

3. Balance your hormone levels. Your basic hormones are listed on page 00, and you can easily (and inexpensively) measure your hormone levels cheaply without a doctor.

4. Exercise regularly, even if that only means taking a thirty-minute walk every day. Exercise is vital, and it is best to have a balanced workout of aerobics and resistance training.

5. Fast one day a week, drinking only water from dinner to dinner. Fasting is the most powerful healing method known to man. Join our monthly Young Again two-day fast during the last weekend of each month. The fasting calendar is at youngagain.org.

6. Do not take prescription drugs, except *temporary* antibiotics or pain medication during an emergency. There are rare exceptions, such as type 1 diabetics on insulin.

7. End any bad habits such as alcohol, caffeine, nicotine, or recreational drugs. You don't have to be a saint, but you do have to be sincere.

References

Chapter 9

1. *Cancer Research* v 59, 1999.

2. *American Journal of Clinical Oncology* v 20, 1997.

3. *Hubei Yike Daxue Xuebao* v 19, 1998.

4. *Journal of Urology* v 163, 2000.

5. *Journal of Urology* v 169, 2003.

6. *Prostate* v 47, 2001.

7. *Journal of the American Medical Association* v 276, 1996.

8. *Journal of Urology* v 144, 1989.

9. *Cancer Epidemiology, Biomarkers Preview* v 6, 1997.

10. *Journal of the American Medical Association* v 265, 1991.

11. *Prostate* v 27, 1995.

12. *Journal of Clinical Endocrinology and Metabolism* v 82, 1997.

13. *International Journal of Andrology* v 25, 2002.

14. *European Journal of Cancer* v 20, 1984.

15. *Steroids* v 89 (2014)

16. *European Urology* v 50, 2006 and v 65, 2014

17. *Experientia* v 35, 1978.

18. *Drugs & Aging* v 17, 2000.

19. *Prostate* v 3, 1982.

20. *Journal of Sexual Medicine* v 11, 2014 and v 12, 2015

21. *Prostate* v 4, 1983.

22. *International Journal of Cancer* v 108, 2003.

23. *Journal of Urology* v 170, 2003.

24. *World Journal of Urology* v 31, 2013

25. *Acta Endocrinologica* v 81, 1976.

26. *Journal of Andrology* v 21, 2000.

27. *Cancer Causes and Controls* v 8, 1997.

28. *Prostate* v 12, 1988.

29. *Journal of Urology* v 196, 2016

About the Author

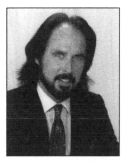 *Roger Mason* is an internationally known research chemist who studies natural health and longevity. He has written ten different unique and cutting edge books about his findings. He sold Beta Prostate® in 2011, walked away from radio and TV, and formed a charitable trust. He lives with his wife and dog in Wilmington, NC, where they run Young Again Products. You can get his free weekly newsletter, read his books, and his three-hundred articles for free at www.youngagain.org.

Index

Other Square One Titles of Interest

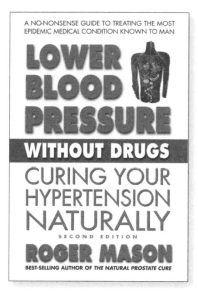

A NO-NONSENSE GUIDE TO TREATING THE MOST EPIDEMIC MEDICAL CONDITION KNOWN TO MAN

LOWER BLOOD PRESSURE WITHOUT DRUGS

CURING YOUR HYPERTENSION NATURALLY

SECOND EDITION

ROGER MASON

BEST-SELLING AUTHOR OF *THE NATURAL PROSTATE CURE*

Lower Blood Pressure Without Drugs
SECOND EDITION

Curing Your
Hypertension Naturally

Roger Mason

Over 65 million Americans have high blood pressure. Although prescription drugs may effectively treat this problem, they have potentially dangerous side effects. Fortunately, natural alternatives are available. In this updated edition of *Lower Blood Pressure Without Drugs,* best-selling author Roger Mason provides a proven nutritional approach to lowering blood pressure safely and naturally.

The book begins by explaining what hypertension is, what causes it, and how it is diagnosed. From there, it goes on to describe how a simple diet, rich in whole grains and low in fat, can improve both blood pressure and general health. This is followed by chapters that address such key topics as the best nutritional supplements to take; which exercises are most effective; how to maintain hormonal balance; and, just as important, how to overcome poor dietary and lifestyle habits. *Lower Blood Pressure Without Drugs* can be your first step towards safely and effectively improving your health.

$9.95 US • 128 pages • 6 x 9-inch paperback • ISBN 978-0-7570-0366-0

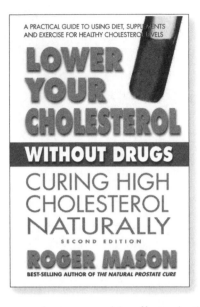

Lower Your Cholesterol Without Drugs

SECOND EDITION

Curing High Cholesterol Naturally

Roger Mason

According to the American Heart Association, high cholesterol is the leading cause of coronary heart disease, which continues to be the number-one killer in North America. While millions of people take prescription medications to lower their cholesterol, the fact is that these drugs often have very dangerous side effects. In this updated edition of *Lower Your Cholesterol Without Drugs,* best-selling author Roger Mason offers you safe and natural alternatives to effectively lower your cholesterol levels. He does so in a no-holds-barred manner, separating the fairy tales from the scientifically valid truths.

Roger Mason begins by explaining cholesterol—what it is, how it is measured, and why high cholesterol is so dangerous. He describes how poor nutrition contributes greatly to poor health. Just as important, he explains how a balanced, nutrient-rich diet can naturally and safely lower cholesterol. You will learn which foods to avoid and which can provide important benefits. You'll also discover how to read food package nutrition labels, and you'll become familiar with natural supplements that can help lower even genetically high cholesterol.

If you think it's time to achieve a healthy cholesterol level without using risky prescription drugs, you have come to the right place. Doing so is neither complicated nor expensive—it is simply a matter of knowing the simple steps to take. With *Lower Your Cholesterol Without Drugs,* you will have the solution in hand.

$9.95 US • 128 pages • 6 x 9-inch paperback •
ISBN 978-0-7570-0367-7

The Natural Diabetes Cure

SECOND EDITION

Curing Blood Sugar Disorders
Without Drugs

Roger Mason

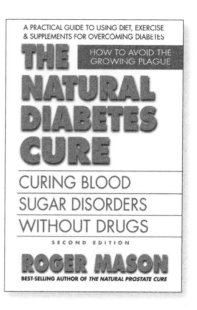

Nearly 20 million people in
North America have diabetes, and
each year, the number continues to
grow. Diabetes can be easily prevented
by simply maintaining a healthy
balanced diet, but many people don't
realize the serious consequences of that
routine trip to their favorite fast food
restaurant. Fortunately, best-selling
author and health advocate Roger Mason
is here to help with his updated edition of *The Natural Diabetes
Cure.* Here is a simple, yet effective nutritional approach to
preventing and combating diabetes.

The Natural Diabetes Cure begins by explaining how diabetes
develops, its major causes, and the severe health risks
associated with this metabolic disorder. The book then details
how a balanced diet of whole grains, fresh vegetables, and
healthy fats not only helps improve overall health and well-
being, but also prevents conditions like high blood pressure,
obesity, and insulin resistance, which can lead to type 2 diabetes.
Additional chapters discuss nutritional supplements that can
help regulate blood sugar, and explore important topics such
as hormone balance and exercise.

Living with diabetes does not have to be a life sentence. You
have the power to free yourself from this disorder. *The Natural
Diabetes Cure*—with the very latest information on natural, safe,
and effective treatments—will show you how.

$9.95 US • 128 pages • 6 x 9-inch paperback •
ISBN 978-0-7570-0369-1

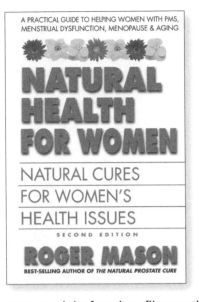

A PRACTICAL GUIDE TO HELPING WOMEN WITH PMS, MENSTRUAL DYSFUNCTION, MENOPAUSE & AGING

NATURAL HEALTH FOR WOMEN

NATURAL CURES FOR WOMEN'S HEALTH ISSUES

SECOND EDITION

ROGER MASON

BEST-SELLING AUTHOR OF *THE NATURAL PROSTATE CURE*

Natural Health for Women

SECOND EDITION

Natural Cures for Women's Health Issues

Roger Mason

Every day, millions of women are subject to their changing hormones, which play a vital role in the functioning of a healthy body. When hormones are not produced in the proper amounts or they are not in balance with one another, a number of health problems can occur, including premenstrual syndrome (PMS), pelvic inflammatory disease (PID), menstrual dysfunction, fibrocystic breasts, and menopause. Symptoms of hormonal imbalance can range from mild cramping, irritability, and food cravings to hot flashes, night sweats, and mood swings. Even serious conditions and diseases, such as osteoporosis, arthritis, diabetes, premature aging, and cancer can result. Standard hormone replacement therapies are often used to maintain proper balance; but they can have dangerous side effects. Roger Mason, in his newly revised *Natural Health for Women*, offers safe and naturally effective alternatives to help keep hormones in balance.

Natural Health for Women begins by first explaining how the body produces and uses different hormones, and how hormonal levels change during a woman's lifetime. It goes on to discuss the various hormone replacement options, as well as safe, natural alternatives. A healthy diet and exercise program is also presented as an effective preventive measure against hormone imbalance. Other topics include natural cures for osteoporosis and arthritis, steps for maintaining good breast health, and how to avoid a hysterectomy.

Hormones do not have to control your life. With *Natural Health for Women*, you can learn to effectively maintain their proper balance safely and naturally.

$9.95 US • 160 pages • 6 x 9-inch paperback • ISBN 978-0-7570-0368-4

Testosterone Is Your Friend

SECOND EDITION

Understanding & Controlling One
of Nature's Most Potent Hormones

Roger Mason

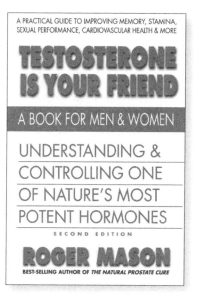

A PRACTICAL GUIDE TO IMPROVING MEMORY, STAMINA, SEXUAL PERFORMANCE, CARDIOVASCULAR HEALTH & MORE

TESTOSTERONE IS YOUR FRIEND

A BOOK FOR MEN & WOMEN

UNDERSTANDING &
CONTROLLING ONE
OF NATURE'S MOST
POTENT HORMONES

SECOND EDITION

ROGER MASON

BEST-SELLING AUTHOR OF *THE NATURAL PROSTATE CURE*

Although testosterone is considered a male sex hormone, what many people don't realize is that this vital hormone is also present in females. For men, it is mainly responsible for stimulating and controlling characteristics that are considered "masculine," like muscles and hair growth. However, for both sexes, low testosterone levels can cause countless health problems, including memory loss, anxiety and depression, osteoporosis, increased cholesterol levels, weight gain, sexual dysfunction, and infertility. While testosterone supplements are available, most are ineffective, and some are even dangerous.

In the updated edition of *Testosterone Is Your Friend*, author Roger Mason presents the latest and most effective natural treatments and supplements to help raise testosterone levels. The book begins by looking at how the body uses testosterone and how this hormone functions differently in men and women. Later chapters examine how testosterone deficiency affects various health conditions. In addition to presenting safe treatments for elevating testosterone levels naturally, the author also explains how simple it is to test the levels yourself.

It's time to re-energize. With *Testosterone Is Your Friend*, you will have the latest information on how to increase your testosterone levels safely and naturally. By following the advice within, you can improve not only your sex life, but also the overall quality of your life.

$9.95 US • 128 pages • 6 x 9-inch paperback •
ISBN 978-0-7570-0371-4

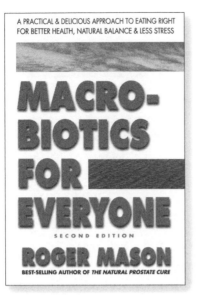

A PRACTICAL & DELICIOUS APPROACH TO EATING RIGHT FOR BETTER HEALTH, NATURAL BALANCE & LESS STRESS

MACRO-BIOTICS FOR EVERYONE

SECOND EDITION

ROGER MASON

BEST-SELLING AUTHOR OF *THE NATURAL PROSTATE CURE*

Macrobiotics for Everyone

SECOND EDITION

Roger Mason

In today's busy stress-filled world, maintaining a healthy, balanced diet can be a constant struggle, and making the right food choices is not always a priority. We may be considered an educated society, yet we seem to be blind to the fact that our diets are typically unhealthy— low in whole grains, legumes, and fresh produce, and high in processed, fat-laden, sugary foods and beverages. This places us at risk for such serious health conditions as heart disease, arthritis, diabetes, and cancer. The truth is that practicing good dietary health is not as difficult or as time-consuming as people might think.

In his new, concise guide, *Macrobiotics for Everyone,* best-selling author Roger Mason makes healthy eating fun and, most importantly, easy. Expanding upon the Japanese macrobiotic tradition, this book offers a diet that is not only creative and less restrictive, but also delicious and satisfying. The book begins by defining the macrobiotic philosophy and tracing the history of the macrobiotic movement. It then concentrates on simple yet practical ways in which you can integrate the macrobiotic diet into your life. Later chapters explore essential issues such as the use of natural supplements and the importance of hormone balance and exercise. As an added bonus, a section on reducing stress through meditation is included.

A balanced diet and lifestyle can both prevent illness and serve as a powerful healer. With *Macrobiotics for Everyone* in hand, you will learn the simplest and most effective ways to achieve both balance and good health in your life.

$9.95 US • 124 pages • 6 x 9-inch paperback • ISBN 978-0-7570-0372-1

Your Blood Never Lies

How to Read a Blood Test
for a Longer, Healthier Life

James B. LaValle, RPh, CCN

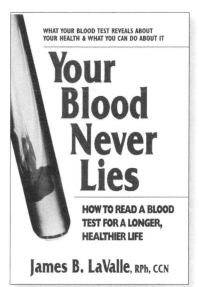

If you're like most people, you probably rely on your doctor to interpret the results of your blood tests, which contain a wealth of information on the state of your health. A blood test can tell you how well your kidneys and liver are functioning, your potential for heart disease and diabetes, the strength of your immune system, the chemical profile of your blood, and many other important facts about the state of your health. And yet, most of us cannot decipher these results ourselves, nor can we even formulate the right questions to ask about them—that is, until now.

In *Your Blood Never Lies,* Dr. James LaValle clears the mystery surrounding blood test results. In simple language, he explains all the information found on a typical lab report—the medical terminology, the numbers and percentages, and the laboratory jargon—and makes it accessible. This means that you will be able to look at your own blood test results and understand the significance of each biological marker being measured. To help you take charge of your health, Dr. LaValle also recommends the most effective standard and complementary treatments for dealing with any problematic findings. Rounding out the book are explanations of lab values that do not appear on the standard blood test, but that should be requested for a more complete picture of your current physiological condition.

A blood test can reveal so much about your health—and *Your Blood Never Lies* gives you the information you need to understand your results and take control of your life.

$16.95 US • 368 pages • 6 x 9-inch paperback • ISBN 978-0-7570-0350-9

The Acid-Alkaline Food Guide
SECOND EDITION

A Quick Reference to Foods &
Their Effect on pH Levels

Susan E. Brown, PhD, and Larry Trivieri, Jr.

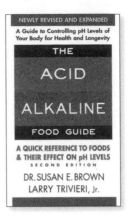

The importance of acid-alkaline
balance to good health is no secret.
The Acid-Alkaline Food Guide was
designed as an easy-to-follow guide to
the most common foods that influence
your body's pH level. Now in its second edition, this bestseller
has been expanded to include many more domestic and
international foods. Updated information also explores
(and refutes) the myths about pH balance and diet, and guides
you to supplements that can help you achieve a pH level that
supports greater well-being.

$8.95 US • 224 pages • 4 x 7-inch paperback • ISBN 978-0-7570-0393-6

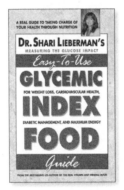

Glycemic Index Food Guide

For Weight Loss, Cardiovascular Health,
Diabetic Management, and Maximum Energy

Dr. Shari Lieberman

By indicating how quickly a given food
triggers a rise in blood sugar, the glycemic
index (GI) enables you to choose foods
that can help you manage a variety of
conditions and improve your overall
health. This easy-to-use guide teaches you about the GI and how
to use it. It provides both the glycemic index and the glycemic
load for hundreds of foods and beverages. Whether you want
to manage your diabetes, lose weight, increase your heart
health, or simply enhance your well-being, the *Glycemic Index
Food Guide* is the best place to start.

$7.95 US • 160 pages • 4 x 7-inch paperback • ISBN 978-0-7570-0245-8

**For more information about our books, visit
our website at www.squareonepublishers.com**